D1524190

Shelved

A *Memoir* OF
AGING IN AMERICA

Shelved

A *Memoir* OF
AGING IN AMERICA

Sue Matthews Petrovski

Purdue University Press
West Lafayette, Indiana

362.61
PETROVSKI

Copyright 2018 by Purdue University. All rights reserved.
Printed in the United States of America.

Cataloging-in-Publication data is on file at the Library of Congress.

Cloth ISBN: 9781557537898
ePDF ISBN: 9781612495088
ePUB ISBN: 9781612494999

Front cover art, *Nana Shelf Portrait,* courtesy of designer Darragh Casey.

Darragh Casey is an Irish designer maker currently living in London. His MA project, *Shelving the Body,* addresses the typology of the shelf with a physical consideration for the figure, subverting our relationships with furniture and reassessing the idea of the "user." Recognized for its alternative design thinking, *Shelving the Body* has been widely exhibited, collected, and commissioned. His book of the same title, produced with Soapbox Press, documents the project from initial MA research to recent commissions.

Casey has worked with clients including Harley Street Clinic, Camper Shoes, Central Saint Martins, *Vogue,* and Van Cleef & Arpels. He also gives workshops and talks around his projects and critical design thinking. Casey currently works as a designer maker at Heatherwick Studio London.

For
Kate Bullock Matthews,
my paternal grandmother
who only began to live
at age sixty-five.
And
to Rudy Petrovski,
my patient, generous husband of sixty-two years,
who has always supported my impulsive ideas.

I dwell in possibility.

—Emily Dickinson

Contents

Foreword

My great-aunt May was, by any reckoning, a remarkable woman. She became a zoology professor in an era when women were discouraged from studying science, wrote a biology textbook that was used nationwide, did research that's still cited by younger scientists, and was, in 1927, one of the first women to attend Indiana University's School of Medicine. She quit medical school when she was hired as an assistant professor at Butler University, a job she held for forty-two years, and she had a long and loving marriage of equals. Aunt May supported her husband, Paul, in his medical practice, and he helped her collect specimens for her lab. They read aloud at night, falling asleep to the sound of one another's voices rather than the television.

In part because she and Uncle Paul were never able to have children, and in part because other family members moved away, I was closer to her than most great-nieces are to their great-aunts; though not as close as I was to my grandmothers, I felt the responsibility. While for years I only visited her on Christmas, when she and her husband moved to a retirement community, I brought my children to have dinner with them once a month and ran errands and, after her husband died, became her next of kin, a surrogate daughter, and power of attorney. When the retirement community said it was time to move her from assisted living to the nursing unit, I was the one who signed the papers and was there on the day she moved. I'm ashamed to remember that I spent more time talking with the administrators at that time than I did with her about the move.

How did I feel about her? Proud, certainly. I knew her story. But if I admit it now, when I was in my forties I didn't really see her. Our conversations were formal. After she moved to the nursing unit, I found myself talking slowly to her as though she were a child, the way the staff and nurses talked to her. Almost daily she was wheeled to arts and crafts activities fit for a five-year-old. This lifelong reader lived now with the television on because the attendants liked to watch TV as they went on their rounds. She had been young once, I knew that, but the only record of her youth consisted of black and white photos turning sepia, photos in which (because of hair and clothing styles) she looked old from late childhood on. Mortal. We crave new styles, I'm half convinced, so we will not be reminded when we look in the mirror of previous dying generations, so we will look to ourselves forever young.

And if her mind was still as sharp as it had been, I reasoned, why didn't she complain? Why did she allow the television to stay on? Why didn't she ask for the music she'd always loved, the books? Of course, I realize now, that I was the one who chose the things to move from her old apartment to her nursing home bedroom. I tell myself that I was busy. She was diminished, I thought, and I was focused on my own trip through this universe.

Still, there were glimmers that the woman I'd been told about for years was the same woman who sat in a wheelchair. Toward the end of her life, as she was looking out the window at the green of the natural world she'd spent her life studying, at the birds on the feeder, she looked at me for a moment and said she didn't understand why she couldn't be of some use. "I still," she said, "have so much to offer to the world."

The system was wrong, and at that moment we both knew this. But I had two children to raise and all I could do was stop by occasionally to see her and feel guilty. It was the one and only time I ever heard her complain.

I tell this story because reading Sue Petrovski's book has allowed me, in retrospect, to see her final years as ones of grace and wisdom, perhaps as a legacy to her family and most assuredly a conscious legacy. It became her final purpose, this wish to cause the least amount of trouble to the young. "I don't want to even put a straw in your path," she said once as she asked for some small favor. Had I read this book before Aunt May's death, I might have *seen* the woman I thought I knew but clearly didn't. I might have understood, in part, the depth of her grief after losing her husband and why she didn't burden me with that grief. Our conversations would have been richer. I missed a chance to learn from her and a chance to give more of myself. I missed my chance to know this remarkable woman.

I began to see how much I'd missed when I went through her papers after her death. I'd been storing boxes of them in my garage. In one box there was a folder of poems and passages of novels that were important to her, passages written on notebook paper and pressed, like the leaves she pressed between waxed paper. There were passages from Willa Cather and Shakespeare and from naturalists like Edwin Way Teale. One of the poems she kept was "A Handful of Dust" by the writer James Oppenheim. The second stanza begins "Handful of dust, you stagger me" and describes the world as it might have been seen by her, as a place "so full of the dead, / And the air I breathe so rich with the bewildering past." The poet sees, in the natural world, the dust of Helen of Troy, of King David, and of the beloved girl to whom the poem is directed. "This is you," he writes, "this of the earth under our feet is you. / Raised by what miracle? Shaped by what magic? / Breathed into by what god?"

To my great-aunt, life was a mystery speaking with voices of the past. "Listen to the dust in this hand. / Who is trying to speak to us?" Oppenheim writes. Listen to those voices, she might have said to me, and tread as gently and respectfully as you can. Or rather, as she did say to me, I now realize, in her actions.

We look at a group of elderly people in wheelchairs, with canes and walkers, and we don't see the individuals they not only once were but still are. In *Shelved,* Sue Petrovski speaks for all our elders as she asserts her individuality and, most importantly, lets us hear her voice. Like my great-aunt, she does not complain. She does not put a straw in our path. She makes close friendships, a home, and shows us how her husband, in the early stages of dementia, is helped by the social and communal lifestyle. Even pointing out that a retirement community is communal in the way that moving into a college dorm is communal is a useful insight. The analogy changes the lens, brings with it the possibility of growth and change.

You will find useful information about aging and decision-making in this book, but ultimately it's the voice of this graceful writer, and her insistence that despite being "shelved" a person can continue to live a life of meaning and purpose, that will change your perceptions of aging and of the aged. Like me, you may look at the faces of the aged, or your own inevitable aging, differently. And perhaps it will bring about change in the way we treat the elderly.

We need voices like Sue Petrovski's in the same way we need the voices of all the marginalized. Our imaginations are so insular and so limited. You can look back through all the ages you've been and empathize with the hopes and fears of a twenty-year-old when you're sixty, but the reverse is seldom true.

Or you can read books, books that expand your perception, your empathy for yourself and others. The book you hold in your hand now is a testament to hope and to the human spirit. I read this book in manuscript form, and I haven't been quite the same since.

SUSAN NEVILLE
Demia Butler Professor of English, Butler University,
Author of *Sailing the Inland Sea*

Preface

Something is wrong with the way in which we currently view elders and their care. I discovered this a bit late in life, and not until this thing called *growing old* began to affect my existence. Did you know that we elders in America are generally viewed as useless? Pondering this has made me wonder if I am truly as useless as I am led to believe.

Shelved is the story of what happens to two ordinary Americans, my husband and me, when suddenly made aware that we are now part of the aged generation and, henceforth, considered to be on the shelf, America's home for most persons over the age of sixty-five. (Sixty-five? Really? I'm eighty-five and still causing trouble!) My intent in writing this book is to draw attention to what research and specialists in caring for the aged are saying about the positive value of this last third of our lives, and how what they say disagrees with the way in which our culture has chosen to view anyone over the age of sixty-five. I also try to inform the reader about how it feels to leave a home one has lived in for forty-seven years and move into a large senior independent living center, with all the adjustments to communal living and the corporate design of said center that are required. We were not ready for this move, nor were we prepared for the fact that we were now considered old, has-beens, over-the-hill, and were even infantilized.

Younger friends have challenged me. "I don't see it that way," "I don't shelve seniors," "I don't treat Grandpa like that," they say. And I am the first to admit that not every person fits this profile. But it is possible that we all are unwitting partners in ageism, the most unrecognized bias in America.[1] We elders are considered an expensive burden, costing millions to maintain, and of little worth to a techno-centered society.

Perhaps this is so, but *Shelved* asks: What would our society be without its older members? Are we of no value after sixty-five? Is our opinion of no worth? Although I have never heard anyone say, "I can't wait to grow old!" I assure you that, contrary to cultural opinion, it is possible to live a purposeful, happy elder life that makes this time rich with meaning. In *Shelved* I share the advantages

I have discovered of these aging years and what I consider to be my job during the time I have left.

In the telling of our story I share some of my friends with you, mostly because they are interesting, but also because they are great examples of value in the elderly population. We older people have learned a lot simply by living our lives—lives full of invention and innovation, years of chances taken and lessons in flexibility. We are insightful, intuitive, and quick to find meaning in the passing parade.

The oldest of the baby boom generation have already crossed over the line from adulthood to elderhood, joining my generational cohort, known as the "silent generation." I wish you all a meaningful journey. I am sure that the boomers—all seventy million of them—will demand more of this final time of their lives, their health, and their care than previous generations have required or received. I would so like to be around to see what they can make of this last third of their lives. Let us hope that they will be aware of their value and determined to make something of these years.

> It is lovely to meet an old person whose face is deeply lined, a face that has been deeply inhabited, to look in the eyes and find light there.
>
> —JOHN O'DONAHUE, *ANAM CARA*

An important PS… I don't want to leave this preface without thanking Kelley Kimm, senior production editor for Purdue University Press. She should be included in any accolades this work may receive. Without her help this would be only an old lady's meanderings. With her help it has become a study in aging. Kelley, your help has been invaluable.

ONE

An Unexpected Page of Life

I hope it does go on and on
forever, the little pain,
the little pleasure, the sun
a blood orange in the sky, the sky
parrot blue and the day
unfolding like a bird slowly
spreading its wings, though I know,
saying it, that it won't.
(SUSAN WOOD, FROM "DAILY LIFE")

In the corner of my mind reserved for precious childhood memories is a vision of a book of unbelievable magic. As I open its pages, a small village appears, rising from the two-dimensional into a delightful three-dimensional paper world—the extraordinary, our reality, emerging from the ordinary. In my aging mind I see Brigadoon, rising to reality, destined to disappear once again, speaking to us of the inescapable passing of our life.

We all know that life has margins. Once we are an adult we know that, and we have no choice but to accept that what we have been given is a precious, unexplainable point in time. Here I am, poised at the edge of this eleventh-hour moment, just before life's inevitable disappearance. Perhaps these are the most precious moments of all, given to us at a time when we are most susceptible to needing a glimpse of the nuances and small wisdoms of being.

By looking within a bit, we may gain a sense of the enchantment of the life we have been given, or what we might call the poetry of our existence. This last chapter, which has seemed so unyielding, such a permanent, unbending force, is probably going to be short, and so we must decide quickly: What shall I do with these months or years? How do I live this miraculous moment in time? How can I see it as magical and vigorous and not as a time of unhappy tears?

Contrary to what our culture teaches, that old age is a sad and dreary time to endure but not enjoy, many oldsters I know would deny that these years denote the absence of all the joyful pages of life. Granted, old age is often a time of added illness, and we probably spend more time at the doctor than we did at thirty-five, but until end-times come, most of us have no trouble laughing and enjoying these gifted years. With a bit of effort on our part, and a show of wisdom, this precious time can be to us a beautiful, rich, meaningful interlude between now and then. It offers a different kind of happiness and fulfillment than we found earlier in our life, but it can be sincerely rewarding, and its tentative quality makes it doubly prized and doubly precious.

That this moment is the only one we know that we have for sure gives it an uncommon quality. I am eighty-five, and I sense that this is such a moment in my life. Please join me as I share this time with you. Rather, let me clarify: I am unable to tell you what aging is like if you haven't been there, but I want to tell you what I am learning from the experience.

It is not to our benefit, however, that much of Western society sees old people as needing to be shelved, a tagline that chronicles our culture's way of registering us as useless, expensive, and a difficult obligation. That said, Medicaid costs for seniors are expected to soar. According to Natalie O'Donnell Wood of the Bell Policy Center, Colorado alone "can expect significant growth in age-based Medicaid expenditures—from $1.04 billion in FY 15–16 to just over $2.325 billion in FY 29–30, an increase of more than 100 percent" based on recent projections from the Colorado Futures Center. Wood states that the CFC "lists two reasons for this projection—growing enrollment and growing health care costs for this age cohort."[1] Added to that, according to the US Government Accountability Office, about half of all households aged fifty-five and up have no retirement savings at all.[2] Such concerns need to be considered and ideas engendered to deal with these discrepancies, instead of simply cutting benefits for this growing group of Americans. The shelf for the oldsters of 2030 may become very wobbly if we wait till 2029 to consider solutions.

However, recent research tells us that it is possible, and even likely, that our elder years have hidden value and worth for both ourselves and others, even as we gradually begin to lose skills and health. The experts also inform us that we have some control over how rapid this loss will be. *Shelved: A Memoir of Aging in America* is my attempt to unearth the truth about this time of life.

Should I make the effort to present as complete a human being as possible to my world? Or, rather, fold my tent and prepare for Brigadoon?

I need right here to let you in on a little secret: I honestly like myself better now than I did when I was younger. These years and my experiences have deepened my understanding of myself, my life, and my view of others. And living in our new retirement community (which I like to call "Planet X"—more about that later) has changed some of my attitudes, making me, I think, a more complete person. My secret motivator has always been hope—hope that I will not die until I am happy with the me that I am. I still have some unfinished matters to attend to (which may be obvious to those who know me), and I wish not to leave until I like myself a bit more.

So let me begin my story ...

As though coming out of a dream a few years ago at eighty, I woke to find that I had long since opened this unfamiliar page in life's book called "old age." I must admit that I hadn't recognized much slippage before this rather late date, but it kind of makes sense considering the reputation age has among my cohorts. One doesn't brag about getting older. One doesn't even admit to it until forced to. Instead, one tries to "think young." I just hadn't thought much about being old. I didn't feel old; I felt good! I was lucky enough to still be able to get around well and participate actively with both young and old friends and keep conveniently busy.

I have since found that it is usually a sudden illness or trauma that wakes one up to the fact that life is gradually ebbing away. But my husband and I had not had any such serious moments and thus had little reason to "think old." Our time of awareness came when suddenly (or so it seemed) my husband began the descent into dementia, while at the same time developing some serious physical problems.

As a result, I now find myself and Dear Hubby, also eighty-five, in an existent laboratory of the phenomenon we call aging: Planet X, an independent senior living residence in our hometown. The unexpected and, I must say, unplanned had become a reality. What caused us to leave our home? I sometimes questioned myself: should we have stayed there? But in so many ways this has been a good move that neither of us regrets. The friends we've made here have become very dear. I so value being able to knock on a door and find a friend. And, when needed, a helper is always at hand.

How did this happen to us so quickly? What is it like to grow so old? I am not equipped to give you a blanket description of what aging is like for everyone. I only want to describe what I am learning from my personal experience, from what I see in my friends, and from what I've read.

Younger cynics will claim that intelligence and happiness are not conditions necessarily associated with old age, but the more optimistic souls will want you to know what they are learning as they grow older: there are qualities that keep spirits and souls alive when all else begins to erode. They will tell you that, yes, it is difficult to be upbeat as we lose our physical and sometimes mental charms, but it can be done, and it is often done in spite of. Many of us have suffered painful losses, and we have worked through them. There can be humor, love, happiness, and kindness in the worst of situations, for as many elders have learned, life is not one-dimensional. Living is a complex activity, and happiness and unhappiness, pleasure and pain, peace and discontent are only a few of the moods and attitudes we play with every day of our lives. All life is multidimensional, and this includes people in their eighties, nineties, and even at one hundred—I am a witness.

Are we seniors simply ready for the dump heap, as our youth-centered society seems to think? Have we nothing to offer? Well, read on and decide for yourself.

On the day I finally woke to being old, I had already lost a great many friends and relatives to the great beyond. I cannot help but think that I owe it to those I knew and loved who have already left life behind, the ones who did not have these extra years, to use my remaining years wisely, with an eye toward discovering why I have been given this blessing (or perhaps responsibility) of extra years.

Aging is not a disease. Aging is simply getting older. It begins when we are born and continues until we die. No one has really defined the exact moment old age begins, for we age a little every day of our lives. When are we old? Even at an advanced age we may still have a very important part of our life left. After we reach sixty-five, we may have thirty or more good years left in us. This is about one-third of our life. Most people would consider this a significant time period—too much to simply let it fly by with nothing to show for it. So now the question is, what do we do with this time?

I look around me here and I wonder whether my fellow residents see these years as a gift or a burden. Should I do as some others and quietly watch TV and let time pass? Should I live outside my own life and dwell on my observations and conversations about what others are doing? Should I tell the younger generation what to do (those youngsters who don't bother to ask us for our opinions)? Personally, I think I have better things to do. But the choice of activity is up to each individual, and regardless of how we choose to use this time, we know that it will soon be gone; these are now or never moments.

In the book *The Psychology of Adult Development and Aging,* Ruth Bennett and Judith Eckman tell us that positive attitudes toward aging may be critical for adjustment and survival at this time of life. Their review of the literature showed that negative attitudes contribute to observed maladaptive behaviors among the aged, some of which may result in premature death, and that if people harbor negative views of aging, they may ignore needed services, medical attention, or other assistance.[3]

I am starting to believe that, without meaning to, perhaps because our attitude is maudlin or glum, we are causing our children to think of us as a task rather than a joy. Of course this is a generalized statement, and I don't think it applies to everyone. I believe, however, that there are times when our negativity does affect those around us. Our children watch as our personality intensifies as we grow older. And we are sometimes anxious and display a lack of flexibility, openness, or wisdom. It is easy for us to become more of what we were early in life; if that was pessimistic, rigid, and negative, we may be even more so in our later years, unless we make a deliberate attempt to change our attitude.

Bennett and Eckman also tell us that negative views of aging held by the elderly may reinforce negative views of aging in the young.[4] I believe we must take responsibility for some of the cultural attitudes toward the old. The crotchety, cynical old guy is not a very good advertisement for a buoyant old age, is he? This gloomy attitude can well cause a gulf between young and old, bringing about an aversion that causes the young to disassociate themselves from aging relatives. In fact, it may cause them to become negative and fearful about their own aging. The rejection and misunderstanding of the aged seen in America today, and the unwillingness of the young to plan for their own old age, speak to the current disconnect between generations. This is not a healthy mindset for any society.

We cannot change the inevitable. The only thing we can do is play on the one string we have, and that is our attitude. I am convinced that life is 10%

what happens to me and 90% of how I react to it. And so it is with you...
we are in charge of our Attitudes."

—CHARLES SWINDOLL, *THE GRACE AWAKENING*

Although we oldsters don't talk much about our own aging, except having
an occasional laugh about a fading memory or our lack of ability to work as
hard as we once did, the evidence shows that we think about it a lot.[5] Our
awareness of our own downward slide can be the factor that causes depression
and sadness, but, as with politics and religion, the silent generation keeps it
mostly private.

Here at our newest home there is chitter and chatter and a lot of superficial
discussion and "remember when" talk, and there's a reason for that. Owned by
a corporation, Planet X houses close to two hundred people in what is known
as independent living to distinguish it from assisted living or memory care.
Those of us who now call this home really do not know one another that well.
We have come from private homes, condos, or unsuccessful attempts at other
senior residences, and we are thrown together, helter-skelter, all with needs
and individual quirks.

I call it Planet X because it is so far out of the reality of what life was like
when we were younger. I can't help but think of it as the planet beyond all
planets. Here we seldom talk about the inevitable. We fill time, we converse,
we find friends who can become quite close, and we often "clique up" into tight
little groups who like to eat together, sit together, and feel needed together.
We may joke about wobbly necklines and floppy arms, but death is seldom
discussed. Why talk about it—it's always here. Today at lunch we added up
those who were on hospice care, in rehab, or had passed in the last few weeks.
The total was eight.

We lose friends. And even though the establishment doesn't share a lot of
information, the underground here keeps touch on the absent ones. We mourn,
we wonder, we cry, but most of us accept the inevitable, for that is what it is.
It is the most difficult when we have a friend who has been out walking the
grounds every day, driving her own car and full of life, who falls, breaks a
pelvis, and then develops pneumonia. They call pneumonia the "old man's
friend," but not when it takes a person who seemed to have years left to live.
(Dear Reader, when one is old, falling is to be avoided at all costs: a slip on

the slushy ice, a tumble, a broken pelvis … these can lead to an unhappy end for someone our age.)

For all of us, aging is a white jigsaw puzzle with blank pieces, requiring us to do our best to turn away from the gloomy attitudes that abound while trying to maintain a curious, creative, upbeat attitude about our own life. We well know that before we can sort out life's subtleties it can all be over, so the need to set about living, friending, and being is now. I know I must truly live every day I have left.

It is common knowledge that aging is something American culture tries to ignore and dreads and dreads dreadfully. We don't do aging well. We have been looking in mirrors since we were very young, watching for that first gray hair or that first wrinkle. We want to avoid it, pluck it, cover it up, Botox it, and tell it, *Stay away from my door, thank you very much.* Most books on aging preach a doctrine of how to stay young, and late night TV proudly promotes skin cream that promises to make you look like you're thirty-five again. I've read articles on women who, out of desperation, have had multiple plastic surgeries, blind to the ultimate futility of their actions.

Are we all so afraid of being shelved? Yes, we are. Shelving is labeling; it is telling someone that he or she is no longer of any worth. It is saying: Do not bother us. After all, we younger ones are the important ones. We adults (those of us under sixty-five) are the useful ones. Our ideas are new and yours are old hat. You do not work, you do not earn, you cost us money, and most of you are useless. To that last sentence: yes, yes, yes, and no. We are more important than is recognized. What happens to a society that acknowledges no past wisdom and sees its elders more as infants or a problem than as purveyors of knowledge and experience? In our cultural blindness we forget that the adults of today are the elders of tomorrow. What will tomorrow's aged inherit from the shelved generation of today? Will they, as some of us currently are doing, find meaning in these last years—meaning at both the individual and the societal levels? I know for certain that they won't enjoy feeling that they are more a pain than a blessing.

When treated as shelved, we can become cynical, for feeling ignored breeds a sour, entitled attitude that can color our perception of the reality around us. That this "nobodyism" is associated with my age group bothers me. To not be a member of a choice clique is OK; I got used to that in high school. But to be considered of little value in a societal sense is another matter. When does that time come when a person is just a bother? When does the hairdresser start asking you the same question over and over because she didn't listen to your answer the first or second time? Sometimes I see myself sitting on a far distant beach, building a castle in crumbling sand while the world and the "doing people" are somewhere far away, doing and experiencing things they don't share with me.

I think that's one good reason for me to be just where I am. I may be a nobody, but I am where I can spend my time with other nobodies. We are shelved together. And like Don Quixote, I will ride my donkey forever and anon, searching for aging nobodies and telling them that they are not nobodies, but that we have been shelved and it is time to get on their donkey and tell the world that there is life after sixty-five, and that the shelved have something to say. Ride your donkey and show the world that you have worth.

This cultural adoration of the objective world of the busy adult under sixty-five has been most unhelpful to our societal way of life. It has caused us to refuse to consider, or find worth in, either the past or the future when decision time comes. We operate in the moment and on opinion only—not experience or even considered thought. The latest opinion becomes the truth of the moment. *What good does it do to talk about getting old?* our culture asks with a shrug. I take the stance that it does a lot of good. We are wrong, as individuals and as a society, to ignore the aging elephant in the room. It is time for us to face the fact that our society contains the old as well as the young and, instead of avoiding the issue, to open our minds and take a critical look at what this blindness is doing to our culture.

Am I truly on the shelf? Done for? Useless? Is this the way younger people see me? Worse yet, is this the way I see myself? Do I have to sigh and accept whatever society or Medicare chooses to dole out, or can I paint my shelf any color I wish? I shall, indeed, try. I am sad when I hear an elder say that life used to be so good, but (sigh) it's all over and there's nothing to look forward to. Too many of those around me simply endure, perhaps because that is what is expected of us. They tolerate a life half-life because they have accepted society's off-putting ideas about our value.

This loss of respect for our lives, along with how we are viewed, greatly bothers many older people I know. It upsets me to have some younger person say, "Yes, dearie," or act like I have no brain left. Many of my friends here at Planet X have been in positions of reasonably great responsibility, and to now be treated as a child is less than they deserve. For the good of ourselves and our culture, we need to open our eyes. I know I'm not a sight for sore eyes (whatever that is), but young man, I'm beautiful inside. Our world would be better off if you agreed to listen to my thoughts and I agreed to give credence to yours. Together we could rule the future.

Is all the money we spend on Medicare, insurance, and senior wellness wasted on old people? Would it be better if, like the plot of the old movie *Logan's Run*, a sudden glow would appear on our hand, indicating old age approaching, and we would be doomed to death, right there and then? If I am now allowed to grow old in my own time, receiving medical care as needed, the question is why. What good is this time of life for the individual or our society? We are very expensive to keep.

Realistically, when I do open my mind to what the future holds, I would be blind if I didn't see that my years are written in disappearing ink. What I want to do, I need to do now. It is sad to hear people my age say they don't want to be bothered. Soon we won't have to be bothered, but today is the day to care and take up a voice. It is easy to give up too soon. If I do my exercises, I wonder why I bother. If I play games to keep my brain active, I wonder why. Am I kidding myself to think that I can maintain mental and physical health through sheer force of will, exercise, and a positive attitude? Maybe. Maybe not. That is why I'm writing this book. Researching about old age is not going to make my last days any longer—that's in the cards, and in the decisions I make—but the results of what I learn can, perhaps, make this borrowed period of my life happier and more fulfilling, not only for me but perhaps for others as well.

We can use this gift of time to find answers concerning yesterday's events and today's questions, and maybe even find tomorrow's resolve. We can paint a picture, or write a book, or take our grandchild to lunch. Any number of wonderful things. And think of this: possibly by our attitudes and striving we will be able to add something to the social fabric of our society. Conceivably, if we open up the path, younger adults will not look so negatively at their own elder years.

As I have said, what we have now is a society that, for the most part, hates to look at the final few years of their life. This is a harmful mindset that can prevent us from seeing the subtitles, the nuance, the wisdom, the poetic side of life; we blind ourselves from our childhood because we refuse to look to our finale. Where is the depth, the moorings that will keep our culture afloat through coming centuries?

I am convinced that this time in our lives needs to have some purpose and meaning. Why else are we lucky enough to have these years? Looked at with a philosophic eye, old age is, perhaps, a time to grow and develop the self rather than to become a useless and expensive mortal morsel that society must support. Perhaps these years are given us so that we may have time to create a legacy or think some compelling thought that we then pass to a new generation. Maybe I will have the time to begin a project that someone else would need to finish. The beauty of that is that my hand would be in the mix. The question is, what attitudes and choices will help me to be strong enough and wise enough to use this period of my life well? It is important that I discover a mindset that will lift me up and carry me happily through this final drama.

So, let us investigate the American elderly. I'm eager to take this look at myself and my friends and hopeful that within this real look at real people we may find some meaning to our shelf of old age. Is today as good for old people as it can be, as good as we can make it, as good as we deserve? What do the experts say? How does one live each day as wisely and joyfully as possible? How can I still feel a part of the action of a vigorous life, a part of the energy of today? Does it matter? Yes.

I recall that the poet and film producer James Broughton wrote, "You are closer to glory / leaping an abyss / than upholstering a rut" ("Easter Exultet"). Ruts can be comfortable, but addictive. Better to leap and see what we discover in the process.

In addition, we need to convince tomorrow's elders to be practical and plan ahead: to consider how much help they might need, what type of life are they looking for, and how they can find it. And, very important, how they can pay for it. The dollars and cents become more important each year, and care for elderly adults is not inexpensive. As a kind of payback, I plan for my next book to concern itself with those elderly who are unable to afford the elderhood that my husband and I are living. It is a fact that 10 percent of today's aged are living in poverty,[6] and that a large percentage of elderly have to decide between food and medication.[7] This is America. Is this really happening?

However, this is a memoir, and in it I talk about how my husband's and my lives changed when old age came to us, why we live where we do today, and what research has to say about this time of our lives. Nevertheless, the most important question facing me now is, why am I here and what is next? It is the mystery that enthralls and holds us captive.

> Magic; the unthought
> That appears in a reasoned mind
> And gives access to
> Other possibilities
> Of Time and Space.
> Thank God.
> (SUE PETROVSKI, FROM "MAGIC")

TWO

Sideswiped by Age

Nothing you do can stop time's unfolding.
You don't ever let go of the thread.
(WILLIAM STAFFORD, FROM "THE WAY IT IS")

There is a thread each of us follows, and even though the storyline of our life changes, the gist of a personal life, that thread of our existence, doesn't. Most of us can probably identify with the idea of an internal guide that seems to direct traffic in our life. The events and circumstances of our life change with passing years, but we are still the same person, with that same internal thread directing our movements. Somehow, we sense that we won't get lost if we follow that thread, even during times of misfortune and unhappiness. And no matter what happens, we don't let go of our thread. It directs our identity.

That is how it was for us until my husband and I were almost eighty. Then the unexpected happened, and I felt that my life had been sideswiped. It is during times like this that we fear our life thread has been ripped away. We feel that suddenly we are no longer in control, and we finally understand, if we have not done so before, that life is a temporary arrangement. At such a time as this we also discover that the happiness and contentment that we had assumed was almost permanent can be lost in the blink of an eye, or, in our case, at the sight of a yellow streak on a car.

Let me tell you how this happened to us. We were merrily enjoying our retirement. Husband Dear was golfing, playing gin rummy, and voraciously reading; I was teaching knitting at our local yarn shop, writing, and lunching with friends. Between these activities, movies, and trips to see the grandkids, we hardly noticed that we were getting old. Life was good. I could always think of a million things to do, and we spent little time brooding about our age or feeling irrelevant. Actually, we felt like we were in full bloom. Our life threads seemed snug and well attached.

At this time, we were only in our late seventies. We took care of our home (paid-up mortgage) and hired what help we needed to keep life purring. Yes, it took us longer to do things, and yes, our children worried that we might take a fall down the stairs or have some other accident, but life teetered on until, suddenly, we were eighty without much thought. Old? We just didn't feel old. (Personally, as I have said, I still felt like I was forty-five.) And our life was full of a great deal of happiness.

However, I know now that we were foolishly unwise in not keeping a closer eye on our life's unfolding. I guess we thought that things would go on forever, much as they always had, and we pushed old age to the back of our minds. (We Americans are notorious for putting off thinking about old age if we possibly can. When life is uncluttered and going along swimmingly, we are apt to just let it flow.) We were enjoying life as it came, drinking our morning coffee, reading the sports page, and doing the crossword puzzles. Why change all this? As Jill McCorkle says in her book *Life after Life,* "we wait for the bad things that wake us up and shock our systems."[1]

I had had some experience with aging. My father and mother were both gone, and every now and then, on the most average of days, the thought came to me that this was not going to go on forever. Nothing ever does. I can't say I had a lot of fear about aging. I was me, and my life thread seemed tight and well-tuned. It had not sunk in with me that when one is as old as we were, one may have to be ready to reinvent a life. Yes, reinvent a life.

Up to that point we had had no need for much adjustment. We were too busy living, and I did not feel a need for any major repairs in the direction of our life. But looking back now, I realize we were extremely lucky—and a little blind.

There is a lot of narcissism and procrastination in me, and I don't think it is uncommon to avoid thinking about the sag around the midline and the little puff taken as we trudge upstairs. Our personal thread keeps us going, we think, and it can even cause us to be a touch blind. Yes, we had been getting notices from our high schools and college about this and that friend no longer being with us, but even though it hurt to see them go, they lived far away and it didn't seem to relate too much to our daily life. We sent cards or flowers or made a phone call, but our life went on as before.

It occurs to me that there's little problem with growing older if we are healthy and have enough money to keep from eating up our savings. We were not wealthy, but my teaching life had furnished us with a reasonably good pension, and with Husband's Social Security check we were not dipping into our stash. It was fun to be retired and not have to work. It was good to have enough money to hire the grass cut, the house painted, the sprinkler system flushed out regularly, and even a dear lady to come clean every two weeks. As a former teacher, I loved sleeping in and not having to report to the classroom at 7:00 a.m.

And then things changed. My husband had always taken care of the bills and finances, and one day I discovered that he had paid some bills twice. Not to worry, we could fix that. But I began to check the bills more carefully. In the three years prior to this he had experienced two serious falls, both affecting the front of his head, and I had started to see certain changes in his life pattern. I began to wonder if there was some residual damage, but I brushed it aside, not wanting to think about that. Typically American!

Shortly after I started checking the bills, I noticed he was having trouble finding his way to well-known places. I clearly remember the morning he woke me up asking me how to get to his doctor's office, a doctor he had been going to for forty-some years. Along with this forgetfulness, he was doing strange things like keeping his socks in his bathroom sink. Does this sound normal? I guess for him it was convenient. I realize now that he had begun choosing the easy way in every aspect of his life. And little by little, his failure to find his way around was joined by a complete lack of ability to judge time, and later by an inability to consider more than one thing at a time. Yes, dementia is progressive. I must keep repeating that to myself.

Some of the first symptoms were that he would get things out and never put them back. But lots of men do that, I thought. At first, I ignored the fact that I had to repeat things over and over. He never seemed to remember what was said even a few minutes before. But the day he introduced our daughter to a friend as me was the day I had to admit that something out of the ordinary was going on.

My eyes didn't fully open, however, until the day he came home with a bright yellow streak down the length of our car.

"What happened?" I asked.

"What's your problem? Nothing's wrong," he grumbled as he walked away, not pleased with my questioning.

"It looks like you sideswiped one of those bright yellow posts in the parking lot."

"I didn't hit anything." And he was quite indignant that I would think so.

"So are you saying that that post came out and hit you?" An alarm bell went off in my head. What was happening? He didn't even know he had hit something. He had sideswiped that post. No, *we* had been sideswiped. Everything was different as of this moment in time.

I didn't want to see what I was seeing, but I forced myself to consider that my husband's mother and aunt had both died with some form of dementia. I had lived with my mother's Alzheimer's and didn't want to think that I would have to deal with this monster again. I kicked myself for ignoring the signs (deliberately or not) when my husband began this crazy downward spiral that might be called dementia or Alzheimer's or ... I don't think it really needs a name. It just *is,* and it takes over a life. In fact, we who have lived side-by-side with dementia realize that it takes over a family's life. One thinks differently when forced to think for another as well as oneself.

No matter how I wanted to close my eyes to it, it was difficult to ignore a yellow stripe down the side of our car. I had to wake up even though I didn't want to and face what I knew was happening: I would be living in this crazy muddled dementia world one more time. This was a fact whether I liked it or not. My bubble was bursting, and I knew I would have to regroup to face this unexpected and unwanted future. I could no longer deny that age and illness were catching up with us. They were no longer just catching up. The truth was right there in front of my eyes: one bright yellow stripe.

I was not unique in my studied blindness. We all would like to close our eyes to something we don't wish to face. Just pretend it isn't there. Maybe it will go away. Maybe we imagined it all. But that yellow stripe wouldn't go away, and it meant only one thing, which I had learned from volunteering at the Alzheimer's Association: there comes a time when a person should no longer drive. I had to admit it; that yellow stripe could have been a child, and it was dangerous for my husband to continue driving.

Forcing someone to stop driving is one of the most difficult tasks of a caregiver of someone with dementia. But it has to be done. There is no question. No argument. No two ways about it. Other people's lives are more important than the personal anguish of not being able to drive. So, dreading it terribly,

I proceeded to explain to him that I would drive him wherever he wanted to go. I took his keys and waited for the explosion. Closing one's driving years is so tough. A car is an American's key to independence, and I didn't know how my husband would react. In fact, I thought he would throw a raging fit having his keys taken away. (Warning: some persons do.) But he didn't.

My husband had gotten to a place where he didn't react much to any event or change. He was beginning to show an uncharacteristic emotional detachment to much of life. Nothing seemed to bother him, and from this time forward, he seldom seemed to worry or fret about much of anything, unless it meant personal pain to him. Generally speaking, he seemed to be in a kind of limbo. With a frequent smile on his face, he gave the impression of being almost relieved to have me making decisions for him. Even more alarming to me was that he began to get that blank look I recognized so well from my mother and those in her dementia world. Seeing it made me shudder and remember things I had long ago stashed away.

When one is dealing with dementia, there is a time when the caregiver must take charge, and it can be a very difficult thing to do. I had found this to be one of my greatest challenges during Mother's dementia. The child had to become the parent. I remember how guilty I felt when I stole her lockbox key to get to the power of attorney papers that were becoming so badly needed. Now, in this present situation, the wife had to become the parent, and I found that adjustment even more difficult, as well as extremely depressing. From this time forward, everything in my husband's life would be a C-plus. How did you like your steak? C-plus. How was your walk? C-plus. So wretched to never get excited about anything.

I've never been sure who suffers more when the game is dementia. It's probably the family. We have to protect, feed, clothe, think for, and care for all phases of someone else's life, and we no longer have the joy of truly communicating and loving back and forth. It is a burden and the cause of much depression on the part of caregivers. If you haven't had to take on such a role, know that having to think for another is not fun. It is even more devastating to try to feel for another. Is he in pain? Is he sad? Often it's hard to tell. My husband seldom responds when I ask how he is. I have to guess whether he hurts. To me this has been one of the most difficult aspects of this time of our lives. Sadly, to this day there seems to be no cure, no known medication that provides significant improvement. We just shrug our shoulders and make do.

In the beginning, I felt like I was becoming a bossy, domineering wife, and really, all I was becoming was a mother—and a very lonely and sad mother at that. Dementia caregivers will know what I mean. Waking up to caregiver reality is a road to anxiety, and for a while I sank into a crater of desperation: What could I do? I was the only doer and thinker in the home. Husband no longer could do bills or taxes, and he couldn't get the groceries. He just sat on the couch and watched TV, day after day. I hated that. But on the other hand, thank God for TV.

What was hard was that the responsibility for the care of our home and anything regarding our lives was now in my lap. It was up to me to get his meds, worry about him wandering off, and then clean the house, make the meals, pay the lawn man, get someone to trim the bushes, pay the bills, put in a new furnace, clean up the water that came in during a torrential rainstorm, and remind my previously spotless husband to bathe. He who had bathed every morning of his life and done his exercises at 5:00 a.m. no longer wanted to do either, as he would tell me very firmly. Yes, his favorite response had become "No."

For me, the stairs down to the laundry room got longer and longer, and I began to worry about the future—if there was to be a future. I'm healthy now, I thought, but what about a few years from now? What will I do if he wanders? What if he falls? What if I fall? What if he becomes violent? What would I do? I didn't know. I just worried.

One can say don't worry, but when facing the monster that is dementia, we instinctively know that we must be alert, or things can happen for which there has been no preparation. Dementia can destroy a family and cause serious problems for the caregiver, so now was the time for me to find my mental compass and some sense of direction … but I didn't, at least not for a while.

Then one day our thread unraveled even further. He began going to the bathroom every five minutes. I asked him what was wrong, and he gave me a muddled answer. His mind seemed cloudier than usual, so I made an appointment with his doctor, who wasn't in the office. The nurse examined him and did some tests. She was not sure what was wrong, but then suddenly he began to shake violently and gasp for breath. The nurse and I agreed that I should take him to the emergency room.

How lucky it was that we made that decision, for the hospital emergency staff recognized immediately what was happening. Unexpectedly, and without warning, he had gone into what they told me was septic shock. While in the ER he began to shake even more violently and then lose consciousness. Later I learned this was brought on by a severe kidney infection. While he was shaking, I looked up at the pulse monitor and could not believe the way the numbers were jumping around. In a flash, he had several nurses and doctors around him. One took me aside and said they didn't think he would live and asked what type of papers he had signed concerning resuscitation. My knees began to shake. What was happening?

Later I discovered the mortality rate from sepsis at his age is not hopeful. Fortunately, the doctors had discovered that his kidney was severely infected and begun treatment immediately. For about ten days he was in the ICU with terrible residue coming from his urinary tract. They gave him antibiotic after antibiotic and IV after IV. He doesn't remember anything that happened during this time, but after about two weeks he was sent to a rehabilitation facility where he stayed for twenty more days, unable to walk or even move very well.

When he came home he was very weak and relied on a walker. His mind seemed even slower than before, and I later learned that this was quite typical with serious illnesses. His movements during this period slowed to a point that it was almost impossible to walk with him. Some of this slowness has continued to this day. He, who none of us could keep up with, was now walking at the pace of a snail. Even today this is not much better, and therapy has only been temporarily helpful.

All I remember about the next few months are the doctor appointments and blood tests that indicated still another problem, a blood problem that sent him to the Rocky Mountain Cancer Center here in Denver. What next? I thought. It wasn't over. Catheter bag, blood condition, trouble walking, dementia. And if this were not enough, we were told by the dermatologist that he had several basal cell cancers on his face and neck. Some were surgically removed, while others required three weeks of radiation. Doctors, doctors, doctors. Illness after illness. Bills, bills, bills.

After much inner panic and, I have to admit, self-pity, I began to know what "till death do us part" meant. Indeed, this is the part of a lifetime that makes it most difficult to not run and hide. At least this was that time for me. I had to sit down quite often and have a serious talk with myself: I could either get a grip on things, or fold up and turn our life over to someone else, or just let it die of neglect.

Recently I asked a friend here at Planet X who lost her husband a few years back when she realized she was getting old. Her answer gave me a big laugh: "Well, I'm eighty-one, but I'm not old. I still get a kick out of seeing those handsome young firemen. How can I be called old?"

I don't know if she was so lighthearted at the time of her loss, but for me, one of the frightening things about what was happening to me during those years was that I still wasn't ready for a C-plus life. I was not experiencing the same physical problems as my husband, and I didn't feel old. What I felt was nothing. How scary. One thing that helped me some was that I had a beginning understanding of dementia and the sundry problems of aging from my experiences with my father and mother. I had found my way out of the Alzheimer's spiral by taking two years in the early 2000s to write my first book, *A Return Journey: Hope and Strength in the Aftermath of Alzheimer's,* and by living through the sadness and emotional highs and lows that Mother's dementia and my father's death had caused. This provided me with some sane moments when I discovered I must live through it yet again, even though panic was my partner much of the time. Experience can be a terribly difficult but good teacher. I was trying to accept that I was still a wife, but I was now also a mother to this man. To anyone who has not lived through this type of crisis, this must seem a strange thing to say, but those who have experienced what we experienced know what I mean and understand the emptiness of such a feeling. Nothingness, emptiness, and aloneness: this was what I was feeling.

The only possible future I saw was filled with pain. I truly believed that our joy was over, suddenly and completely. Was this what our old age was going to be like? All the fears of myself and my culture welled up in me in these moments, and I had no partner with whom to discuss what was happening to us. I am a great fan of *Winnie-the-Pooh,* written by A. A. Milne, and I recalled a favorite scene:

Piglet sidled up to Pooh from behind. "Pooh," he whispered.

"Yes, Piglet?"

"Nothing," said Piglet, taking Pooh's paw. "I just wanted to be sure of you."

I needed for someone to hold my paw and tell me everything would be OK.

Nostalgia and sadness consume my thoughts when I look back at these months. We want to stuff our hurt, but it engulfs us, haunts us. I covered up my pain with eating, but all I felt was anger at myself for reacting to my feelings in such a childish, unsatisfactory way.

I remember few details about this time, but I do remember looking through our wedding pictures. There he was, handsome in a white dinner jacket. Both of us with stars in our eyes. Life had now taken a 180-degree turn. No more fun, I thought. Looking back now, I realize I had much to learn. Here I was, eighty years old, and I still expected fun and joy to be presented to me like gifts tied up with a silver ribbon. I hadn't learned, even at this age, that fun and joy are self-taught and come from within, not without. Sometimes it takes guts to find joy—like looking at the handsome young fireman at a time when this seems like a silly thing to do. Why not!

I'm glad that I had the sense to not just give up, lock the front door, and turn on the gas. Like all of us, I have this life thread, and I had always had a fairly positive outlook, although at that time I felt only numbness and anger and a sense that my world was turning upside-down. Basically, I love life. I had always acknowledged how precious it is, and that one does not give it up without a damn good fight. Suggestions from my daughter, son, and my inner self convinced me to pick myself up and start looking for solutions to the emptiness I was feeling. My daughter and son both gave me such good advice that it made me very sure we had raised wise children. And it helped so much to be able to share this passage with them. The part I didn't like was that I knew all of what was happening hurt them as much as it hurt me. At such times as I have described, strange ideas can enter our tender world and give us direction. Funny, but true: I thought of something Lou Grant said to Mary Richards on the Mary Tyler Moore Show: "You've got spunk." I'm southern Indiana Scotch-Irish, and I was hoping that heritage would protect me. I prayed that we would get through all this, but it would take me some time to feel solid enough to call forth that spunk. At the time, I was too busy doling out meds, changing linens, and still having moments of both panic and pouting.

I must admit, for a while I seriously hoped someone would tell me what to do, because I surely didn't know. This is what happens, I thought, when one doesn't look ahead. For heaven's sake, we were eighty. What had we expected at eighty? No . . . sorry, that's not quite right. *I* had to get my head together and decide what *we* wanted to do. I had forgotten, for a moment, the new reality: *I* now had to think for us both. If I continued to wring my hands and not move, others would decide for us. I just had to find my spunk.

Plans, however, would have to come later. Looking back, as I said, I remember little of these first dark months: I remember a lot of washing, visits to get his catheter changed, trips to the radiologist, going to the grocery store, and I remember trying not to think much about anything. These first weeks following the breakdown in our happily-ever-after were the victim of my depression and shock. Trips to doctors were taken, meals were cooked, errands were run, but it was as though someone else was doing all of this busy work while I was ensconced within my brain. Thinking, thinking, thinking. Why had I not prepared for a time like this? Why had it floored me so? Why (even) was God punishing me? Yes, I even blamed God for my lack of preparation for old age. Poor God. He didn't deserve it. I was the one who had thought that the bugaboos of illness and age would not dare sit on my front porch.

I later realized that there are various reactions to the thought of old age and the sundry illnesses that often usher it in. One can cry, take to one's bed, and let family and society deal with you and it. One can give oneself over to old age. As one friend said when I asked him what he was going to do this afternoon: "As little as possible." This is another response to ageism. One can mentally retreat, going through the motions of life but totally separated from reality for a period of time. Or one could be prepared and ready to go on with life at a different level when Old Man Trouble comes to visit. My friend A. said that she and her husband had been part of a group at their church that visited different senior residences and held group discussions on aging and how to deal with its problems. Now this is being prepared, at least intellectually. Knowing my friend, I know she had emotional needs to deal with as well.

There may be other ways to accustom oneself to the problems of old age, and you, Dear Reader, are free to add your observations. I, however, was a creature of my culture. I didn't want to think about getting old, and as I said, our good health had let us get by with that pie in the sky attitude for many years. No wonder I found myself in such a funk. Like my society, I knew little about making decisions for this time of my life. What does one do in that foreign country called old age—a place for my parents, but not a place I had ever envisioned for myself. Like the society I knew, I didn't want to adjust. I wanted what I had had. The good life.

We can see from my experience that ageism, which is so widespread in our country, has harmful effects on the health of older adults. We don't recognize it as much as we do racism or sexism, but it is there. It is even, as in my case, deep at the core of aging persons, telling us to stay young as long as we can, and when we no longer can do so to give up, hole up, and get on the shelf, bothering others as little as possible. Trouble is, who wants to sit on a shelf? Agers need a paw to grab and the feeling of being a part of it all. So much of my spunk was being used to direct traffic in my husband's illnesses: "Take off your clothes and get into the shower. Don't forget to wash your hair," while silently thinking, "When will I have to get someone to help him do all this?" Whoops, while I'm busy in the bath with him, his hard-boiled eggs explode. I forgot them on the stove, darn it! Phone's ringing: "Yes, oh we're fine. Sure, I'd love to do dinner but don't think we'd better. Maybe later." I had gotten to the point where I didn't want to do anything. It took effort, and I didn't want to be reminded by anyone that we weren't OK anymore. I went silently into my shell, exploding my eggs, washing my sheets, making my trips to his doctors and … gosh, I really don't remember what I did. Isn't that interesting …

I don't assume that all react to problems as I have, but I have discovered that if I don't bring such frustrations and hurt into the open and get a compass to my future, although I can beat back my problems, they will continue to pop up, following me until I find answers and a path to healthy solutions. Gradually I woke from my stupor and my desire to hide. Retread, I began to read, and to talk to friends. I started with some friends from the Alzheimer's Association:

"Dad got to the point he was eating Brillo pads."

"You think that's bad? My dad got lost while they were on a trip and they didn't find him for days."

"You've got to watch. Mom tried to climb over the deck railing."

I had forgotten just how bad dementia can be. Because I had experience with Alzheimer's, I knew a lot of the horror stories, but since my mother's death they had always happened to others. Such stories were important for me to listen to now, however, for they made me aware that whatever I planned for our future had to take dementia into its design, and whatever we did we had to plan for the progression that is part of the disease. When dealing with mind things, the future is always different from the present. What if even some of the things my friends told me about happened to us? Where could we live together that would give me the help I needed to deal with our altered life?

I could live in our home, but could I find adequate help? Could I bring help in or would it all be up to me? Would I have to place him in what is known as a memory unit? Could we afford it? Questions, questions.

What I am saying is that I needed to plan for the future as well as the present. I needed long-term ideas and goals. I needed to plan as though my husband would someday be very demented and very ill. This could be our future—who knew? My plans needed to include tactics for possibilities that were not yet a reality, but could happen; what kind of life design could I find to cover all this? (And frankly, at that moment, I was in no shape to do anything but feel the sideswipe of this newest problem.)

Once I began to wake up and study our situation, I discovered that my attitude and habits would have a lot to do with our survival and future happiness, which helped me to find some control once again. As my friend group agreed the other day, whenever we are sideswiped by sadness, grief, or even tragedy, we just have to work around the clinkers in our paths. Everyone has them, and this is true no matter what age we are.

Clinkers are OK. T. S. Eliot is quoted as saying, "If you aren't in over your head, how do you know how tall you are?" The fact is, in any confrontation, we go into the fracas, whatever that may happen to be, trying to make decisions that we can look back on as wise and well timed. That's the way life has to be lived, I have found. On the edge. At least this is true of my life.

Dear Reader, you may dispute this, but I stand by my opinion. I have since learned something that I wish I had realized back in these black days: the tough moments in life can make us the kind of person we've always wanted to be. If handled well, they can help us find love, kindness, and wisdom within ourselves. If we are proud of the way in which we handled the toughies, we grow. At this point I am only putting this forth as a possibility, one which I will speak of in a later chapter. The point I need to make here is, I was learning and I was growing, even though I didn't like what was happening to us.

In these dark moments I began to realize that there are lots of alternatives in life. Our aging life can appear as a beat-up old car that chugs through a crossroads, hiccups a few times, and either comes to a halt or the cylinders start firing. Or we can learn that there are alternative choices that will make the trip more enjoyable and even longer lasting. I wasn't ready for the halt part yet. I have always personally considered life to be so spectacular that, regardless of what we have lost, or how our backside bulges, I hope we can be here just a little longer. Just a wee bit more time, please. We have stuff to do, and we want our partner with us, doing the future as well as he or she can. In this frame of mind, I began to grab hold of my life's thread and take reassurance in what had directed me in the past; we say a prayer, cross our fingers, move on, and hope.

I reminded myself that aging isn't a disease, even though society may see it as such. It does, however, come with cells that no longer turn over quickly and a body that has lived through all sorts of emotional and physical traumas. Yes, we elders are well used, even well abused at times. But we have lived through other travails. We are survivors, and if we can heed the advice of medical inquiry, perhaps it will show us that maybe, just maybe, there is more time left in which to find joy in a life that can be put to good use.

I hope it is apparent from my mistakes and my unprepared state that it is wise to recognize that we will die, and that if we live long enough, those last years will be better if we know what to expect, and if we are able to pay for what we need. That is so important. I always nod in agreement at those TV commercials that urge a lifetime saving fund that will become a personal retirement fund. Too many of America's old are living at or just above the poverty level (not to mention the 10 percent living below). It costs money to be old. My advice to younger adults is to make the necessary adjustments as you age, put some money in the bank, and think a bit about how you want to spend these latter days. I was so glad when trouble hit that we had enough of a backlog to give us some choice.

An added bonus is that boomers are apparently not as blind to the problems of aging as me and mine are and were. They are beginning to assert their influence on how they want their future to be. For example, according to Gay Hanna and Susan Perlstein, authors of *Creativity Matters: Arts and Aging in America,* this expanding group is offering those in the creative fields an extraordinary opportunity to transform the experience of being old, giving meaning and purpose not only to aging but to the community at large.[2] Thanks to the boomers, it is possible that we are now beginning to see older people for their potential as well as their problems. I became quite motivated to study this research, particularly that which describes some of the new attitudinal investigations of aging people.

Be of good cheer. Attitudes and knowledge are a-changing among the medically sophisticated, if not in society at large as yet. We are beginning to see a tiny crack in the attitude that elders are useless, and studies (discussed in later chapters) are confirming the worth and health of the American aged. Things are looking up. Aging is starting to be viewed not as a horrible prelude to death but as a time of ripening and creativity. Instead of dried-up old fossils leftover from adulthood, we are now being considered by some as essential to a well-rounded society. Let us be hopeful.

Ultimately, we survived my husband's illnesses, and yet we were not as we were before all this happened to us. No one ever is. Our family talked seriously with me about changes that were needed in our current lifestyle. Husband was now up and around, but weak and not the same man. I was happy to be with him, however, because he was still a smiling, happy old man. And although I remained responsible for most aspects of our lives, I wanted us to be together. Still, we had to face the fact that neither of us will get any stronger or more able. So, what now?

Girls, you've got to know when it's time to turn the page.
(Tori Amos, from "Northern Lad")

THREE

Choosing Our Tomorrow

Mockingbirds aren't content to merely play the hand that is dealt them.
Like all artists, they are out to *rearrange* reality. Innovative, willful, daring,
not bound by the rules to which others may blindly adhere, the mockingbird collects snatches of birdsong from this tree and that field ... recreates
the world from the world.

—TOM ROBBINS, *SKINNY LEGS AND ALL*

Life is made up of improvisation, and like the mockingbird we sometimes have
to invent a new song from this field or that tree in order to find the strength to
move into a new act of our life. We are at a loss to recognize what harmful
influence will materialize that may cause us to have to recreate our world,
but sadly, when this adjustment becomes necessary, fear is our most common
response and the motivator of last resorts and lost causes. Regrettably, instead
of logical thought, it is fear that can initiate a panic reaction, causing us to
hunker down and avoid taking any risk, choose the easy path, or go into fren-
zied action with limited information. How do I know this? Because I'm an old
woman, and experience is not a new thing for an old woman.

No doctor was able to tell me specifically what would happen next
with my husband's dementia, or what various other physical problems he or
I might develop. Nor could any doctor tell me how soon this or that would
happen—who knew? Because of my experience with my mother, however,
I knew that I probably could expect my husband's dementia to worsen over the
coming months and years. Just how quickly was the big unknown. Couple this
with the fact that because of our age and his various physical conditions, our
children were urging us to make some changes in our lifestyle. ("Do you think
you're safe here now, Mom?") At first all I could think of was: Where would we
live? What to do with the multizillion objects we had collected in our lifetime?

Mingled with our kids' concerns about the common dangers that old
people face (the stairs, the stove, the shoveling in winter) was my own sense

of not being quite as able as I once was; it was no secret that I probably would not become stronger as I aged. Face it, Mom and Dad were getting old. We (or now, I) could no longer be Don Quixote flailing at windmills and ignoring that old bugaboo called age. Too bad. It was fun while it lasted. Unfortunately, I have always been one to close my eyes to things I didn't want to see, but this was not a pristine time to do so. This was a time to consider carefully and logically the next chapter of our lives.

Playing on that concern, our son sat down and dialogued with his father, suggesting that we move to a place where we could get help when needed. His father, in his semi-demented state, resorted to the negative as usual and didn't hesitate to answer, "Over my dead body." Well, that was that. My previously agreeable mate had made his opinion known. So, what does one do? His dementia was obviously one of the factors causing him to contest any change. His world was becoming narrower and narrower, and as his dementia grew, he clung to his little sureties and anything that would make life easier.

As I mentioned in the previous chapter, he had developed the habit of saying no, regardless of the question, and he was growing fonder of his C-plus world. Like a small child, as long as he had his cookies, ice cream, and root beer, the rest of the world was forgotten. Turner Classic Movies became his world, and it was somewhat worse in the evenings. It's called *sundown syndrome.* Dementia patients can be relatively sound all day, and then around four o'clock in the afternoon they can begin doing and saying strange things. With Husband it was, and still is, more that some days are better than others. I can do no wrong on days one, two, and three, but watch out for day four. He has never been physically violent, but he's moody. Very moody.

This was obviously a time in our lives when I needed to improvise: like an artist—like the mockingbird—how could I rearrange our reality without destroying the love and closeness we two had shared all these years? I love Husband, but it troubled me that both our lives might be determined by his fade into dementia. I knew I would not be content living in a C-plus world. I just knew I wouldn't.

Although I had to take a few pills for this and that, I still felt well, but when we are in our eighties, who can count on continued good health? All of this convinced me to begin exploring and unearthing what I had neglected to inquire about in earlier years concerning the old person scene in America—to finally snatch a bit of birdsong from this tree and that. This old bird wanted to search other trees to find a new home, one that would allow me to go beyond "playing the hand that was dealt." My experience with Mother's illness had shown me that this is my life, too. But the problem many caregivers have is determining how to manipulate their lives so there is a place, some contentment, and some care for both.

Years ago, when the time came to place my mother in an Alzheimer's unit, I explored options, but I knew a lot had changed since then. That was in the early 1990s, and mostly the choices were to stay in your own home, live with the kids, or go into assisted living, an Alzheimer's unit, or a nursing home. Some of us were reminiscing yesterday about our grandparents' and parents' fear of having to "go to a home." Families who placed their old folks in these "hellholes," as one elderly father had called them, were often looked down upon. (What? You didn't take Aunt Louisa into your own home?) I remember so well my great-grandma in her print dress, heavy socks, and black shoes sitting in that empire-style oak and black leather rocker in my grandparents' home. It seemed to this young girl that that was where she was supposed to be, and I never heard a cross word between her and Grandma. Great-Grandma Hart would take me into her neat-as-a-pin bedroom and show me her "buryin' clothes" and how to make crepe paper flowers. My grandma loved her mother and would never have considered not having her in her home. After all, when my grandmother's first husband died young, her parents took her and her two children into their home. Families took such moves in stride in the 1920s.

But that was then. I had a sense of dread when I thought about the type of care we might receive today. Memories came back to me of how it had been when I looked for a place for my mother ... I couldn't forget the smell and obvious minimal care offered in a great number of those homes. I was not ready to place myself or my husband in some of the places I remembered. So many old folks sitting in rows in front of the TV, or lying, seemingly unattended, in bed. As I saw it, in most of those homes the plan seemed to be wash 'em, feed 'em, and hope they don't need any more attention. (This of course was my own prejudiced view. But we all have a right to our prejudices, as long as we recognize them as such, don't we?)

Most of the patient care was provided by the aides, and nurses seemed glued to their pill-pushing trays, seldom looking at the patients as they shoved their meds. I know this is a generalization, but I saw it often enough when Mother was admitted to know that it did happen, and still does in some circumstances. It has appeared to me a case of the task usurping the attention that the elder should be getting. But perhaps I am expecting too much.

It was only by luck when searching for Mother that something led me to a director of a memory care unit who combined both experience and a warm heart. (Her mother had had Alzheimer's, and this lady understood what demented patients needed.) It's probably obvious to you, Dear Reader, that placing Mother was one of the hardest things I have ever done. I remember so well how difficult it was, standing on our porch ready to help her into the car, when we knew that we were taking her to a home away from her home. And as we stood there she sighed a very small sigh and looked at the world around her. I will always remember that sigh and that final look.

I wanted to avoid that for Husband, and I wanted to be with him as long as possible. But I wasn't ready to live in a locked Alzheimer's unit. Was there another alternative? I had to think this problem out carefully.

Our children were hesitant to push us too much for a decision and kindly repeated several times, "We want you to do what will make you and Dad happy, but what will that be?" At one point I muttered some reply, I don't remember what, but basically something like, "I'll think about it."

It would be an easy, quick decision to simply stay where we were. I could take care of our home, as I had for years, and I could take care of Husband, too. Oh, but I forgot: things have changed, now. Did I really want to take on the task of mothering the home and the husband? I have never been a willing sufferer. I am not a martyr. I'm getting old. Did I really think I would be able to care for this old house, cook meals, do the washing, clean up the basement every time it rained and water came through the windows, arrange for all the repairs needed in our old house, decide on what kind of new heating system we would need, and take care of a husband with dementia and several other physical issues?

As I said, I am not a martyr, nor am I unrealistic. Perhaps I could cope with all this responsibility as strong as I was at the time, but could I count on continuing good health? I remembered what I had learned as a volunteer with the Alzheimer's Association: caregivers often develop illnesses and go before the loved one does. The strain of caring for another takes a heavy toll on an aging body.

Mixed with our children's concerns was my sense that I was not quite as able as I once had been. I liked to think I was just as spry as ever, but when I was honest with myself, I had to admit that it was harder get up when I weeded the garden, I was tiring out much sooner than I liked, and I took meds for blood pressure and a thyroid condition. Would I be happier if I had less housekeeping, washing, and cooking to do? Yes, I knew I would be. I found myself dreaming of a place where I would have the free time to do things that interested me, meet with others with common interests, and just take care of my husband and myself. No, I was not willing to be a sacrificial victim, and although I was more than willing to care for Husband, I needed a place where I could care for me as well.

Rumi, one of my favorite philosophers, wrote, "Lovely days don't come to us. We must walk toward them." Nobody was going to help me improvise this new life that I imagined in my dreams. I was now responsible for the happiness or unhappiness of us both, and the thought of that was exhilarating but also very worrisome. The idea of a new start, a new environment to investigate, and perhaps some help caring for Husband brightened me. It was something to look forward to after the months of working to get him on the road to recovery.

Later research showed me that Rumi was even scientifically correct: it is good for older persons to have something positive to work toward, hopefully some happy days. We all know what a positive word or look can do when our world seems ready to collapse. Still, to many women of my generation, decision-making about life-changing moves can be frightening. Would I make a mistake and move us to a place that might cause us unhappiness in our final years? Would I be able to deal with all the emotions that would come into play if we decided to leave our home of forty-seven years? Would Husband adjust? (Obviously, this was a huge question mark.) And, let's face it—would we be reasonably happy, and if so, for how long? There was always the possibility of staying where we were and making adjustments to our living quarters, but at considerable expense in this old house.

I was suddenly the captain of this aging ship, and someone had to make decisions regarding where and how it was to sink or swim. Questions flooded my brain. For one, would we be happier simply staying where we were for as long as possible? We had friends who had made this very choice. But the danger is that one sometimes stays just an inch too long and the house takes them over. I couldn't help but remember an acquaintance who stayed in her home after her husband became demented. They did well for a while, but one sad day the wife was found at the bottom of the basement stairs. Her husband had covered her with a coat but had not been able to think to call 911.

I am a list maker, and so I began thinking on little pieces of paper. Post-its were made for me. I checked off some of the basics we would need: a place to sleep, eat, make friends, and get help if we needed it. Check, check, and check. We both might eventually need physical therapy, nursing care, and exercise opportunities. And from my mother's Alzheimer's I had learned that dementia patients require certain key environmental options: a place to live without too much challenge, social contacts that are not too stressful, and small tasks and jobs they can do that make them feel useful. Later I might have to worry about wandering, but that would be in the future, I said with my fingers crossed.

The answer to the dilemma of what choices to make when one is old varies with each person, as it should. Many of us cling to the surety of past memories and huddle close, cozily ensconced in our beloved home. Others are like my friend who had been a caregiver to her husband for ten years, then honestly came to the place where she said, "I knew I needed a place that would take care of me." I agreed. Having lived with dementia before, I knew I needed a home—a place where my heart and mind could grow; someplace warm, welcoming, and where I would have friends and help to lean on if I needed it. Was there such a haven or heaven? I prayed there was.

One of my personal reasons for even considering leaving our home is evident in one of the notes I wrote: "Help! I can't do this." Here we were in our early eighties, and I had not yet admitted that I just couldn't be a good caretaker for my husband and also keep up with all the home responsibilities I had handled so easily in the past.

I secretly dreamed of a place where I would be able to spend my free time on projects and activities that tickled my fancy and still be able to do what I needed to do for Husband. *Why couldn't we get what we both needed?* I asked myself. It was a relief to admit that I had my own desires.

Moving isn't easy at any age, but one doesn't do it at eighty unless there is a good reason. We had that reason; I was ready. Selfishly, I thought that was reason enough. It would be work for all of us, but if we waited, closing the house and selling everything after we were gone would be an even more difficult task for our children. In spite of Husband's harsh *"No!"* this move had to happen.

What has kept some of our friends in their own home, or living with children, is their mental image of moving to an old folks' home—some depressing place that is perhaps medically sound but cold to the touch. A nursing home environment comes to mind. As I mentioned, our generation has memories of senior places that were not so pleasant. Some of us remember while searching for a place for Mom, smelling the urine in the carpets and looking at old people lined up watching TV. If given that choice, and only that choice, I would have stayed in my home and taken my chances. The thought of moving into hopelessness is grossly unappealing. Our mindset can be shaped by these disagreeable recollections from the past, and it is hard for our generation to believe that pleasant, caring places exist. We often have to be convinced, and some elders who have such ingrained ideas, but who are unquestionably in need of care, may have to be forced to move from a home that is no longer safe, even though it is much better if the elder agrees to the move.

I'm happy to report that we are beginning to see some forward-thinking senior homes. A few are quite elegant, some are very expensive, and others are well appointed, have a modicum of care when needed, and a homey atmosphere. My friend A., who had been living alone, shared why she moved to our present home, Planet X: "Life is too short to babysit a house. I'm having a ball here." Why not? She kicks up her heels at Friday's happy hour and eats meals she didn't have to cook, enjoying them with a variety of friends. Loneliness is another reason elders choose to move: My friend B.'s husband died, and she felt so very alone in their big old house. Others move to senior homes because they want to live closer to their children but don't want to buy another house.

I considered that perhaps I needed to find a professional to help me make a decision. There are numerous home care groups willing to help seniors. Some organizations are free, while others charge. My advice would be to choose such help carefully and not limit yourself to just what you are told by one group or another. I got on the computer and looked for an organization, or persons, that would be able to give me some in-depth information on various choices and residences with the hope that they would have ideas I hadn't considered. However, after checking with a couple of popular organizations, I found that they couldn't tell me anything more than I could find with an internet search. A wonderful resource is the Seniors Blue Book, which provides one of the most complete listings of senior homes and senior help I could find. The printed guides are free and even tell you minimum rents and what is offered in each residence. Although the guides are not available for all areas of the country, the website (www.seniorsbluebook.com) is a great resource no matter where you live.

There was one group I called that I wish I hadn't. They simply regurgitated information I could find on the internet and then proceeded to notify most of the possibilities they had mentioned and had them contact me. The phone rang and rang, but all that accomplished was confusion and wasted time on the phone. Another thing that bothers me is that some counselors hide behind the "we cannot take sides" rule if you ask their opinion apropos which place they would recommend. Caution causes them to hesitate to recommend any one residence.

Consider carefully what information you need. One thing I wanted to know was what home services are available through Medicare. My most valuable resources in my search were my computer and my friends. Many of your friends may have gone through this search with their parents or friends, and I found that talking to friends and checking out their suggestions saved hours of personal searching. A careful search takes time and effort, I found, but by reviewing our finances and getting help from reliable sources, we managed to avoid some of the problems older people face, such as getting care that doesn't really care, or paying more than we have to for a new place to live, or being fed lies about what we would get for our money.

I relied most heavily on my instincts and conversations with my daughter, and if you can smell a rat fifty feet away and know how to ask the right questions, I would still recommend a personal search. I must admit, my best instruction came from my sixth sense. In talking to others I found that this sixth sense seems to be the most valuable home-hunting tool for many.

And I had another rule of thumb: When interviewing for various teaching positions during my career, I had always carefully considered the personality and philosophy of the principal. The mood of any establishment usually flows downward, I have found, so I looked to the top to see if I would be happy working or living within the personality and philosophy I found there. Every place we toured, we asked to see the director of the residence, not just the sales person.

The problem I have since discovered, however, is that once you are in a residence, the leadership can change often as a natural process of promotion or resignation, invariably causing a shift in the direction and mood of the place. We've had four executive directors here at Planet X in the three-plus years we've lived here, and all have elected to run things their way, interpreting corporate guidelines as they personally see fit. In many cases the corporate owners are the "principals" that one needs to investigate. What is their reputation?

Getting a new director can be confusing to residents. I just heard that we are getting a new director. My reaction: Oh dear, what will this new one consider important? It's like starting a new grade with a new teacher.

Another point before we go on: scams out there today are a real problem for the elderly. This is a bit off the subject, but please don't send money to lawyers in Canada to secure a place in an inheritance. Don't give your Social Security number to some stranger on the phone. Our elderly neighbor did that, and her entire bank account was taken. Also, widows, do not become cash tickets for younger men. A long-term friend without children fell for that one and, whoops, there went her money. This is a time to deal only with someone you trust, and to be wary of trouble lying in the weeds. I don't want to sound overly suspicious—there are a lot of good, kind people in the elder care industry—but double-check the information you get.

Older persons look at this late move in their lives in such different ways. We had been in the same spot for forty-seven years, and I saw this as a time to freshen my outlook, as well as an opportunity to change Husband's C-plus view of life. I needed to feel enthusiastic about our future, and a new move and the possibility of new experiences and new friends did that for me. Even at eighty, I still needed activities, people to see, and places to go in my life.

As I write this, I realize that this can be a major roadblock for dementia caregivers. How does one design a life that supports the condition of the one while also satisfying the desires of the other? It is so easy to feel trapped and frustrated, but I encourage caregivers to continue to underwrite their personal needs. We were fortunate to find a place where we both could feel content, and I encourage anyone facing a similar situation to continue to search for a solution that considers both persons, even if it takes some time to do so. In such a case, the solution may be as we found it: a place where I would have limited work caring for our apartment and meals, could take care of Husband's needs, and could still find a place for me.

Considering Husband's present opinions and expected response, my children and I stealthily set out to do the legwork necessary to find a solution. I felt like a traitor, for Husband and I had always made all major decisions together; however, I knew that this time I would have to do the deciding. Those who have lived with a partner for many years will know how I felt. There are times in life when couples must adapt: marriage, parenthood, and now, dementia. Each new stage brings with it a feeling of uncertainty, of teetering on the edge of we know not what. Each is a time of decision. If we make the wrong decision, we could probably change it, but if we turn our decision over to others, we live what they would do—not what we might choose. Ergo, I wanted to take care in making this decision I knew I was making for both of us. If it was a wrong decision, so be it.

If you've ever searched for a door in a totally dark room, you know how I felt at this time. I reminded myself that not only had I survived all past stages of my life, but I had helped my parents through their very last adjustments. I had learned a lot and thought I should be able to manage this as well. I had our children to help, and what a great help they were.

We often act from what we see as mistakes of past generations. Part of my decision to move was based upon a memory of my mother. I can still see her standing at the patio door, sighing out of loneliness, but unwilling to make any positive changes in her life. Early in her dementia she was so unhappy that it made me feel singularly frightened about my own old age. Remembering her unhappiness, I now had to shake myself and keep in mind that I am not my mother, and that this is a different time. I was willing to fight to keep from living my final days in gloom and doom, as I had seen her do. These are the thoughts that kept me looking for something more, something to look forward to. My daughter will tell you that I'm not always this brave and farsighted, but this is my book, so I will try to paint myself in a positive light. The search was on.

With this tentative decision to move in hand, the first concern I had was to understand our financial picture. Like many women of my generation, I had left a lot of the financial decisions up to my husband, but now Husband was unable to handle things, and who else was there to do it? I could have found a financial adviser, or turned it over to the children, but I am a do-it-yourselfer and thus felt that I needed to get my own hands on the figures. And I knew I needed to check with a lawyer to see if our will and all those power of attorney papers were still relevant, considering we had filled them all out over twenty-five years ago. Now was the time to have them checked for usability.

I needed to figure some things out. How much could we afford to spend? What kind of dream home would our savings and investments provide? How much rent could we afford? Old age isn't cheap—a truth that was reinforced over and over during our search. Few of us want to be a burden on our children, and in order to avoid this, I had to know if we had enough in savings and investments to care for us until we died. What kind of living could we afford and still not spend everything and have to rely on the next generation? No dreaming or pie in the sky solutions at this stage would do. I had to know the facts, so I divided the total value of what we had saved and invested by the largest number of years we were likely to live and asked myself: Do the plans we wanted to make sound reasonable and realistic? Would our monthly income from my pension, his Social Security, and our investment dividends cover our expenses? Yes, I considered inflation, as well as growing medical costs and increases in our health insurance. I even considered that investments in mutual funds and stocks might dwindle or at least not earn anything. I tried to account for the worst that could happen. After I totaled all this, I looked at the value of our home.

If we sold our home, we could add the money we received to what savings we had. But how much was it worth? Friends were saying that it was a real buyers' market in our part of town, so perhaps for many reasons it would be a good time to sell. Click, click. I added the possible money from the house into our total reserve. (Many elders today are living in senior residences on the profit they are getting from the sale of their homes, which have been selling at relatively high prices.)

Of course we will all have different answers when evaluating our financial future, and what is most important to you might not be what's most important to me. Given that, here are some of the things I stayed awake at night fussing about:

1. How much will different living choices cost us?
2. What do we really need in terms of space and available help?
3. Where would we be happy? To endure is not enough. I am not willing to settle for just OK, and I don't think anyone should be unless it is absolutely necessary.
4. Where can we get medical help and find well-conceived activities? Bingo isn't enough.
5. Where is this paradise I wanted: meals, housekeeping, places to exercise and walk, socialization, activities, and help when needed? I had decided

that these things were almost a necessity if we were going to go through the work and anxiety of a move at our age.

With all these thoughts and figures bouncing in my head, I began to look at alternatives. I have kept some of the lists I made, and looking back at them now, I am a little proud of the manner in which I navigated this terribly important time in our lives. Here are the eight options I came up with:

1. We could remain where we were. This would necessitate the expense of taxes, insurance, lawn care, upkeep, and what promised to be extensive work on our older home. It also would require money for groceries, clothes, and so forth. However, in today's Medicare world, in-home care would be available for most of our personal medical needs. Insurance companies have begun touting home care because it is less expensive than hospitalizing the old, and currently about 75 percent of elders prefer being cared for in this way. We could spend our money on home upkeep and even bring in meals and other services. It might work for a while, but what about when Husband's dementia grew worse?

2. I could remain in the home and place Husband in a memory care unit. What would that accomplish? I asked myself. Probably nothing. We would have to live apart, and I would still have all the work and expense of our home, plus the very high costs of a memory care placement. And he had not yet progressed to the stage where he needed such intensive care.

3. We could both move into a senior apartment. There are many fifty-five-plus places out there. There would be no help, nor food service, but we would have lower living costs, and service and medical care could be imported. However, we would be pretty much on our own and couldn't count on interesting social activities any more than if we had stayed in our home. All we would have is less space and less upkeep on our home.

4. We could move in with our children. *No.* I immediately crossed this off the list, except in a case of emergency. Looking back, I am glad I made that choice. It isn't that our children aren't caring, but it's a living arrangement I wouldn't want to burden them with unless it was absolutely necessary, and it was not. We are lucky to know that both our children are there if and when we need them.

5. We could get some kind of trailer and put it on our kids' property. They even have what are called Granny Pods now, with a small bedroom, kitchen, and bathroom. These pods can be moved to wherever they are needed, and they even have a built-in ability to report medical information. Then, there are those tiny houses we see on TV. *No.* These present the same problem as #4 and probably would be too small for two old people.

6. We could move into a senior trailer park, a move touted in a recent issue of *Time*. For example, if you want to "move to Florida and play golf, go to the beach, enjoy life," life in a trailer can make it possible.[1] One would have sociability, and entertainment, for a fraction of the cost of life in some other ways. This could be a possibility, but I'm not sure that this would be a good solution for Husband and me.

7. We could move into a house in a neighborhood that had been renovated to accommodate six to eight needy elderly. I knew little about these and would have to investigate.

8. We could both move into an independent senior home of some sort. These sprang up after my parents' illnesses, and I knew little about them. I did know that meals and housekeeping were furnished in some, and I learned that most have accident alert systems, and that we would have many other persons our age in a structured social network. Sounded good, but were there some drawbacks? Yes. They are expensive, and in independent living, only certain kinds of help are available. Or this is what I was led to believe. Later I discovered that this is changing with our modern care communities. From the present Medicare point of view, home medical care, if you qualify, is available even if your home is an apartment in a senior care facility. Watch this space, however. We all know how the future of Medicare sways with the political tides.

In recent years, as independent residences have added personal care attendants to provide assistance with hygiene, nutrition, and a long list of daily tasks (as well as companionship), they encourage a belief that elders can stay longer in an independent environment, and in some cases even when they need hospice care. These residences describe it as moving the care to the patient rather than the patient to the care. This is now commonly referred to as aging in place, and there is even a national council for it: the National Aging in

Place Council (http://www.ageinplace.org/). The one question I had about moving to such a place was whether they would accept my husband with his dementia. I discovered that there is no dementia care available, except that offered through occupational and speech therapy service providers, and that is minimal, but dementia has its stages and types and in many cases, with help, dementia patients are acceptable in some of these independent homes.

In my new mulish frame of mind, I called our children and said, "Let's get busy and see what kind of senior home we can find for Dad and me. And, oh yes, I think we should sell the house." I heard a sigh of relief on the other end of the line.

As we get older, it is easy to become self-absorbed, and we are not always aware that our aging efforts seriously affect our children. They do worry. Over the last few years, when I would call my daughter or son before eight o'clock in the morning, their first response was, "Is everything all right?" I hate to admit it, but we have become the bomb ready to explode, and our children have become alert to possibly being needed at a moment's notice. I know this because I remember being there for my parents.

Thus began our search. Telling Husband I needed to do some shopping, I went with my daughter to visit several independent apartments and cottages on senior campuses, gathering information on pricing and what was available in each place. I began a list (yes, one of my lists again) of the various amenities and prices at each location: name of residence, phone number, available units, price; meals, laundry, cleaning—how often and how much; parking, storage, maintenance; activities, health care available. Last but definitely not least, I listed how much this would cost us each month. It sounds like a lot of work, but I was choosing a home for what I hoped would be the rest of our lives. I had to ask a lot of questions. I think you will find, as I did, that what they say is the price is subject to various additional add-ons: initial deposit of perhaps two thousand dollars or more, pet and parking fees, additional cost for a second person, etc., etc., etc. It's important to get the money involved spelled out clearly from the start.

I found it interesting that many places hide the prices until they have you nailed down with a phone number and other ID. By asking for a price, you become a prospect, whether you want to or not. When you do this, expect many phone calls. If it is as we experienced, you will get more than one offer from some residences. Salespersons for senior housing are astoundingly good at their job, and I found that one has to listen very carefully to what they say and how they say it.

Many older facilities will have residents living there who have moved in over the years under many, many different payment plans. It usually depends on what the financial picture and rental situation was at the time of their move. The more vacant apartments there are, the better the deal one can likely muster. But on the other hand, remember that there may be a reason for those empty apartments. We who shop at stores where the price is usually the same unless it is sale day need to be aware of the bargaining involved in the health care industry. A full house means more income, and the cost to you may depend upon whether they need to fill apartments. Sometimes there are special deals such as a half month's free rent, or extra items added to your apartment such as a new refrigerator or stove, or new window shades. It never hurts to ask.

I might add, don't be afraid to ask questions of residence marketing people, and don't be afraid to have lots of *what if* questions, such as: What if I find the neighbor in the next apartment listens to TV till 3:00 a.m.? What if I need to have food delivered to our apartment from the kitchen? What will that cost me? Where would I do laundry? How much storage is there in the apartment? Could I get a washer/dryer put in my apartment? How often will the rent go up, and by how much? (Count on it going up—regularly. We have found that every January we can expect what seems to us a hefty raise.)

So many questions, but now is the time to ask them. Let me insist that instead of responses such as "Maybe," or "I'll look into it," or "I'll ask about that," you try to get definite answers. There are so many small issues that develop after one has moved in—so many small points that you may wish you had asked about earlier, so many tentative promises that are not in writing that you may not realize later. If you've never gone through such a search as I have described here, I urge you to do so, even if you are not presently considering a move. You will be glad you did. It has opened my eyes to the choices we have for the retirement years. However, be aware that changes are taking place all the time in this industry, and when you begin your own search, you may find a greater or lesser number of options than I have described here.

Touring so many senior homes left me feeling older than I had ever felt, but I certainly became much better informed about senior life. This familiarity can be useful, I thought, if I ever want to write a book about aging. Not only that, we need to keep control of our lives if we can. I have talked to a few residents who let their children pick their new home, and in some cases they have never quite felt at home. It was not their choice.

Finally, after all this, we get to the important part: what did my daughter and I find when we began looking? I was amazed at the selection and variety of senior homes and the possibilities for tomorrow. Elders today are spending their pensions, Social Security, and money earned from the sale of their homes to rent very upscale housing in senior residences, thus making it profitable for investors to provide a wide variety of housing choices for our age group. In our area, new communities are going up as fast as builders can get a loan, and some of them are quite beautifully appointed.

I mentioned that there are senior living apartments that rent to active seniors over fifty-five. These serve the younger elders who are tiring of housework and responsibilities, some of whom have the money to buy services and a new experience for themselves. In my daughter's neighborhood an unused convent is being flipped into apartments for younger seniors. Instead of rentals, the buy-in will be almost equal to what prospective buyers can get for their current home, but the care and upkeep associated with owning a home are largely eliminated. With this money these young seniors are buying recreational time instead of taking care of the house time. Now that I am no longer tied to a house, this sounds great to me.

While we were looking, one of our visits was to a large, attractive facility—almost a small village—spread over several treed acres. It was locally owned, and the buildings included a main building with one- and two-bedroom apartments where meals and housekeeping were included. Across the street were cottages, and farther down the same street was still another newer apartment building. It was a distance apart from the main building and reserved for independent living, with no housekeeping or meals. In addition to independent living and assisted living, the campus had an Alzheimer's unit.

We toured one of their very charming cottages, as well as an apartment in the main complex. The cottages seemed to be a cozy alternative to our present home, and I was smitten. They really were quite nice. The price included rent, utilities, a garage, and two bedrooms. We would have to pay extra for the housekeeping and also for more meals in the dining room. That sounded OK until I remembered how my husband was shuffle-walking: small steps with a cane and so very slowly. Put this together with thoughts of snow in the winter, and I knew we could be trapped in our cute little cottage and have a devil of a time getting to the main building for any meals or other needs. It would have been a good choice for me, but not for the two of us.

The main advantage of this residence was that most of the independent living apartments were somewhat reasonably priced, but of course they were priced without meals and housekeeping. I did like that there were higher levels of care available, including that memory unit, but what benefit would that be at the present time? I would still have to clean and cook, and the social activities seemed questionable and a little outdated. With the assisted living and memory care available on the campus, it was obvious that their philosophy was "move on to another place when you need more care." I listed all the particulars on my inventory sheet and moved on.

We then visited a recently opened, locally owned residence inclusive of independent living, assisted living, and memory care. Three years ago the meals were about seven hundred dollars per month, per person. That plus the apartment would have cost us more than the first residence we visited. I liked the homey look of the place, and I was familiar with it since I had a friend in the assisted living apartments. However, I didn't feel good about the management, and my friend was very unhappy with the food and with their slowness when she needed help. Listening to my inner voice, I felt little empathy with the assistant director, who briskly took us on a short tour before she hurried off to lunch. To top it all off—no dogs allowed. They didn't allow even cute, tiny, good little dogs like our lovable Lucy. So, that settled that; if Lucy wasn't good enough for them, neither were we. I scratched them from our list.

Most senior homes today allow animals. It is a commonly accepted fact that pets are therapeutic for older persons.

I next paid a visit to a third residence. It was close to where my son lived and was a little less expensive than some other places. I can't repeat often enough that in this search it is so important to listen to that small voice inside that says yes or no. The guide was very friendly, the apartments were clean and appropriate, the dining room was OK, and it seemed to have a fitting number of activities for residents. I hesitated. Somehow, although it had everything we were looking for, including a personal care program to help if you needed aid in bathing or dressing, I could not see my husband and me living there. The building was dated, and although it wasn't seedy, it needed renovation and the atmosphere was less than positive—it was stale. Residents sitting in the lobby didn't seem very friendly or happy, and I just had a negative reaction to the place in general. This was an independent living home that was trying hard to be homey and pleasant, but somehow missing the mark. And the salad I had for lunch was wilted and tasteless. Not a good omen.

I'm not sure about the marketing acumen of some of these places. I was given a pie as a parting gift from this last residence, but why they gave it to me I'll never know. When I opened the box I could swear that pie was so factory-made that it was stamped with a serial number. Why would you bless any prospective resident with a gift like that?

Next we looked into independent living residences that require an investment. These mostly ranged from one hundred thousand to two hundred fifty thousand dollars, but some were more. In one, the resident is expected to pay this large sum of money, move in, and then if the resident leaves, or dies, the resident or his or her heirs will get a percentage of the money back, *if* the corporation is able to resell the apartment. There is, of course, the possibility that the corporation may not resell it, and I could not help but think to myself, what if the corporation went bankrupt and, whoosh, there would go our money. Some seniors willingly sign such a contract, but I decided to look further.

One such place was borderline elegant. No, it was really elegant. The entry fee was fifteen thousand dollars, and the apartments cost five to seven thousand a month. It was a gorgeous facility, with paneled walls and tasteful surroundings throughout, but my pencil would get very dull trying to match this to our present budget. I knew I would see our savings disappear all too rapidly in this lovely place. Not only that, I know that I require less charm in my daily life. This was obviously a place for what we used to call "the 400," and socially, I have always been about a 325. I did envy the activities they fostered: trips to the theater, symphony groups imported to play for them, art exhibits, and very creative activities for the residents.

My daughter and I then visited Planet X, which was owned by a national corporation, as most residences are today. We entered a large lobby with a great staircase going up to the next level. The receptionist was oh so pleasant, and we could not avoid the smell of popcorn popping at the boutique to the right of the lobby. A resident was pouring herself a cup of hot chocolate, and several elderly people were walking around, talking and laughing. Somehow I knew this was it. Planet X seemed like a cozy, inviting place, and I began to feel that this might be our new home. Or at least I hoped so.

A charming lady took us on a tour of the building and apartments. The library, theater, and exercise, TV, and garden rooms were the highlights that indicated an active, busy community. On the way to tour an empty apartment, we passed a laundry room and a pool room. The apartment they showed us was small, at least having lived in a house for forty-seven years it seemed that way. However, it had a relatively large living room area and a bedroom with ample space for both an office and a bed. There were two walk-in closets, two coat closets, a linen closet, and a pantry. (Always check the storage in a new apartment. Just remember all that stuff waiting back home.)

Planet X had an intelligent and fun schedule of in-house activities, plus several scheduled trips a week to restaurants and places of interest. The apartment would be cleaned every two weeks, and beds would be changed every week. We would do our own personal laundry, but sheets and towels would be done for us. Here the meals were included, and the large dining hall seemed comfortable but not overly formal. Some of the residents introduced themselves to us. They seemed content and sociable, and one even said she hoped we would join them.

I must add, we were impressed by the friendliness and seeming competence of every staff member we met, and I was especially fond of the setting. I knew our dog, Lucy, and I would be able to walk through the wooded acreage around the property, and as I stood and looked at the entire landscape, I felt a peace that I hadn't experienced in a while. Could this possibly be the place for Husband and me? Had I found a home?

There was one drawback: it wasn't inexpensive. Fearing the worst, the first thing I did when I arrived home was to wrestle with the figures I had compiled to see if we could afford it. I estimated that after selling our home we would have to dip into our savings some each month. How much? I figured some more. We could afford it, but I knew that I had to figure in the rise in the rent that we would probably see each year. It's the nature of the beast. I had never worried much about yearly advances in our pension, but now it would matter more to cover any added expenses. We have since found this to be oh so true: we are now paying 15 percent more for our apartment rent than we were when we moved in three-plus years ago. Some of our friends have not taken this into consideration and are now wondering if they may outlive their backlog.

Beyond the physical facility, I was influenced, I know, by the professed philosophy of Planet X. It was beginning to see itself as the expanded, contemporary version of elder care I had been reading about. It labeled itself as an independent living facility, but in fact it fostered the aging in place philosophy. Physical therapy, home nurses, and occupational therapy, as well as bath and feeding care, transportation, and other helpful aids for residents, could be provided as they were needed. There would even be someone to dole out one's meds or take the dog for a walk. This all came at a price, of course, but if one had to move into an assisted living home to get such services, that would also mean a hefty increase in rent.

Residents could bring in outside help if preferred, and medical services would probably be covered by Medicare Home Care and private insurance. It is a fact, however, that between the federal government and local laws these things change often, so I would once again advise anyone to check this space to get the latest ruling. In our case my financial figuring told me that with Husband's Social Security and my pension, we could manage the rent at Planet X. With the sale of the house and our investments, we would be able to cover clothing needs, food for the apartment, car insurance and expenses, TV and phone, and other incidentals.

As an added bonus, Planet X won our hearts when it welcomed our little dog. The corporate stance was that all its facilities were pet friendly. There were certain rules of course: you must not leave doggie messes on the grounds around the building, and there were to be no dogs in the lobby unless they were only passing through. Only smallish dogs were welcome, but, bottom-line, Lucy was welcome. The company even sent Lucy some doggie treats, and this almost sealed the deal. Now *that* was a great sales strategy.

It began to look like we may have found a place to call home, but I still wrestled with the idea of having to sell our home and cut back on our belongings in order to fit everything into that apartment. I planned to sell the house as soon as possible, but I know this is not the way everyone does it. We have friends here who still haven't sold their home after several months, and others who have rented garages to hold a lot of extra stuff. Perhaps it is comforting to them to think, "I can still go home if I want to."

Early in our married life we moved a lot, and I have always thought that home is in the heart and we can take our memories wherever we go. I knew there would be some emotional moments, but my thoughts at the time were: Why spend money on an aging old house? Wouldn't it better to spend our life's savings on these two aging old people? Before we made the very, very final decision, however, I took another moment to reconsider. While I was deliberating, my daughter, in her winsome wisdom, asked, "What would make you happy?" This was not an easy question to answer, but it was a good way to make the decision. With my known world spinning out of control, I had a hard time deciding. Of course my first choice would have been for my husband to return to normal, but that was impossible.

As I considered her question, I realized how hard it was to believe that we had reached this last stage in our life, our old age. We were old. How had it come so soon? Where had the years gone? I shook my head, wondering why I had not seen it coming and whether everyone feels this way. I answered my daughter by saying, "I think we need to move to Planet X. I think that is where we need to be." "Do it," she replied. And so we did. And more than three years later, I'm not sorry we made that decision.

Of course there are things about Planet X that I would like to change, but we'll talk about that later.

Before we signed the contract, a very nice therapist from Planet X Corporation came to our home and gave my husband a test to see how severe his dementia was. After that we asked for another tour, this time with my husband included. I had no idea what to expect, and my heart raced as I wondered how he might react. The marketing representative took us on the customary tour once again, and since we had warned her that Husband was not in accord with the move, we noticed that she was giving him added attention and even a piece of pie as we toured the dining room. Yet, even with all the inducements, Dear Husband was muttering and growling as he followed. I didn't want to know what he was saying.

Following the tour, we sat down in the marketing representative's office—Daughter, Son-in-Law, Husband, and I—and three of us confronted Husband with the final decision we wanted to make. The poor guy was outnumbered. Grumbling and unhappy about the whole thing, he finally agreed to try it, not realizing the finality of the move, I'm afraid.

It took just two minutes to sign the contract, and, honestly, both of us had only a small inkling of what we had agreed to. I know what motivated me at that time more than anything else. It wasn't courage that moved me to this action, but the possibility of a new, fuller life for us—and for me an end to caring for an old house all alone. Others might have made the decision for other reasons. Regardless of the motivation, to give up a home is traumatic, and I don't mean to downplay the emotional impact of making this move. And let me be clear: no one should make this move unless it is his or her personal choice, or it is absolutely necessary.

A good friend who moved here after us will not go back to see the home she left because it hurts too much. I didn't feel that way then and still don't, but leaving one's home is a very difficult thing for many elders to do. Another friend, whose son forced her to move, hates it here. I've witnessed this reaction several times from those who moved against their will. Me? I told myself I was happy to get rid of the care and upkeep of an older house that would require us to spend a lot of money to make it likable again. I also agreed with a friend here who said, "My kitchen is closed." And so, we moved. Next chapter.

"Go back?" he thought. "No good at all! Go sideways? Impossible! Go forward? Only thing to do! On we go!" So up he got, and trotted along with his little sword held in front of him and one hand feeling the wall, and his heart all of a patter and a pitter.

—J. R. R. TOLKIEN, *THE HOBBIT*

FOUR

Turning the Page

Sometimes memories sneak out of my eyes and down my cheeks.
—Author Unknown

I may be a slow learner, or imbued with a sadly weakened old brain, but gradually I have learned more about this page of life in the twenty-first century. As Mary Oliver asked in her poem "The Summer Day," "Tell me, what is it you plan to do / with your one wild and precious life?" Because I did consider our lives precious, and I didn't want to leave all my wild and wonderful behind, even in my eighties, we made a decision. Well, I made a decision. We would sell our home and move our precious lives to Planet X. Looking back now, I know I felt deeply that this was the right choice, and I still agree that we did what was best for us, even till this day. But I must admit that when I think back on those years of raising our children in those rooms, and roasting marshmallows in the fireplace, I need to have a moment for myself.

When I remembered how lonely my mother had been, I felt that the world of Planet X would be good for both of us in so many ways. Socially, I knew we needed Planet X. I think that was my main motivator. My mother could find no purpose once Dad died, and she had no plans. I watched her pull into herself and saw her life shrivel and die. However, I am not my mother, I told myself once again, and I wanted a different final chapter. I had vowed to find a place where the final years for my husband and me would be as motivating for both of us as was possible, and I hoped so desperately that this move would accomplish my prayerful plans.

It was so important to me that we spend our last years in a place where we would not be alone or lacking friends. Humans exist and thrive in groups, and even in this country of rugged individualists, research shows that we do better if we are a part of a group.[1] This was the influence that pushed me to keep moving forward. I did not want to sigh through my old age, feeling forgotten and lonely as my mother had. It is too easy in one's final years to find trouble to cry over. It is not so easy to develop mental attributes that lead us to find reasons to live and love.

But on with the show. Now we had to deal with the practicalities of this decision. How much does one value the cherished possessions accumulated over all those years of hauling souvenirs home from trips, going to antique shops, and lovingly storing a yellowing wedding dress, carefully wrapped through the years in blue tissue and worn so long ago? What price do we put on boxes of family pictures, keepsakes of baby clothes and tiny little white leather baby shoes, and generally just about all our life seen in material things? I picked up a tiny shoe. Ah, memories. But as I touched its soft white surface, it occurred to me that my memories would go with me wherever I went, and much of the physical stuff of yesterday must stay behind. Our new apartment was not big enough to hold our years of conspicuous consumption. It was only big enough for us and our memories, and Lucy.

We Americans love our stuff. We cherish our stuff. We take good care of our stuff, and we love to buy new stuff. We love to shop, and who can deny that we are terribly fond of the never-ending swag that surrounds us? As children of the depression and WWII, in which we saved the tinfoil off gum wrappers, wound used string into balls, and collected rubber bands with enthusiasm, people in my generation are collectors extraordinaire. We are the generation raised to not complain and to make do with beet sugar and ration stamps, and warned to "waste not, want not." As a result, we complain in a whisper, and we leave our homes and our stockpile of stuff with deeply felt regret and a great deal of wistfulness. I have always been a collector. Be it too many shoes or extra silverware, I collected it and lovingly stuffed it all in closets. Now those closets needed to be emptied.

To be honest, our stuff had gotten to be too much, and I was almost glad to leave this mass of clutter behind. But how to decide what to do with it all? It really had become a heavy burden just to move it around and keep it from smothering us. That I had owned an antique shop for five years after I retired from teaching didn't help the size of our booty. Much of the store stock had been sold, but there remained odds and ends to add to our parents' leavings and to the family stuff we had put away.

I had begun to feel the weight of it, but the question of what to do with it was not an idle one. Give it away? Sell it? Who would want all this stuff? I needed help. We made a small dent in the boodle by encouraging our children to go through each room and take what they wanted. I kept a few favorite pieces: some candlesticks, a pewter plate or two, and many of my favorite books. Our son took Grandpa's antique gun and watch, and our daughter took Grandma's china, glassware, and silverware from two generations back.

The remaining belongings, with the exception of what would go with us, I opted to sell what I could and give the rest to charity. Once that decision was made I was reasonably content, but then suddenly it hit me. All of this turmoil was really just a result of *my* decisions, and here I was, making another major decision without my husband's knowledge: to sell our home of forty-seven years and say goodbye to a large quantity of our possessions. Add to that the fact that he still was unaware that we would be moving *permanently* to a large senior residence where we would be living with up to one hundred seventy people we had never met before in all our lives. Here we were, my daughter and I, behind Husband's back, deciding what to do with fifty-some-odd years of our lives, as seen in this accumulation of antiques and family stuff. I will admit to some disturbing feelings of guilt during this time.

Regardless of the guilt I felt, I had to keep moving and decide what would fit in our small apartment and what we would need in our new life. And then, finally, I had to arrange to sell our home. What was I doing? It was probably just as well that I didn't think too far ahead when we signed those rental papers on our new apartment. I know now that I was relying heavily on that small voice inside, the one that kept telling me, this is right, this is OK.

Decisions, decisions, decisions. Plan to have a few headaches deciding what stays and what goes if you choose to make such a move. There were moments when I walked from room to room, unable to decide anything. I just looked around, and cried. I thought several times about forfeiting the down payment we had made and ignoring any move at all. Other times I looked at all our belongings and tried to decide if we really needed this or that in our new life. That darling little antique pine desk—I wanted it so bad, but where would it fit on the map of our new apartment? And it had a slanted top. Not practical if I wanted to use my computer, and we wouldn't have room for two desks.

The four-poster bed, so high that soon neither of us would be able to get into it, I feared … but it had belonged to my parents. I remembered the night my father chased an invading bat with a broom, and to this day I know which post on that old beauty of a bed was still wobbly from from the vicious swats Dad made with that weapon. Oh dear, oh dear. Could I part with it? Oh dear. The grandfather clock; I loved that old baby even though it couldn't keep time.

So many memories. So many old pictures. So many books. So many age-old thoughts to fight one's way through. Was the future move worth it, or was it best to simply sit and die surrounded by our booty? So tempting.

Getting rid of our stuff and making this move seemed possible but painful, and now looking back from three years later, we did a good job with what seemed to be a difficult and melancholy task. There are still some things I miss, but I calm myself knowing that there wouldn't be any place for more useless stuff. Yes, it's just stuff, and I remember my father once saying, when parting with a favorite antique piece, "I had the joy of owning it, and that's enough. Let someone else enjoy it for a while." I stopped for a moment while writing this, for I suddenly realized that he had relegated the accumulation of stuff to its proper tentative place in his life, and now it was time for me to do the same.

We were fortunate, nevertheless, in that a very nice lady recommended by Planet X helped us determine what furniture would fit in our new apartment, and what would give us the most use. She reminded us that we should try to take items that will provide storage, so we decided on a blanket chest and two chests of drawers, one for my husband's clothing and one for mine. We had boxes of old pictures my mother had collected. There was a large box containing many, many photos of ancient relatives sitting stiffly and wide-eyed before ancient cameras. Who were they? They were complete strangers to me, and obviously so to my children. It was sad, but they had to go, even though my mother was probably looking down and having a fit. We did keep recognizable pictures of loved ones, and they now are stored in boxes on the top shelf, not looked at in recent memory.

This nice lady also helped us make paper patterns of the furniture, and we went to our new apartment and laid our phantom furniture here and there on the floor. It was like building a shadow of our life to come, and I highly recommend doing something like this. Many of our friends brought too much stuff with them, and their small apartments are desperately crowded.

I admit to fretting over this beloved article and that cherished photo during the weeks we had set aside to sort and move, and I tried to tell myself that all this clutter was unnecessary to a happy life, in which people should be our uppermost concern. Anyone who has gone through a wrenching move like this one knows how difficult it can be. The thing that kept me going was the thought that, ultimately, I would have an opportunity to look forward to our future instead of looking backward to our past. It just wouldn't be sound decision-making to let a lot of old things, old stuff, keep us from a hopefully brighter future. It never is.

Keep in mind, however, that our society sometimes makes the elderly feel there is no future, which is one reason many of us cling to what was. I see people cling to things, to people, to habits, and to uncomfortable reactions to change. We have to have something that belongs to us, we say to ourselves, and memories and our stuff are our security. Our culture leads us to believe that this is it—the end of the road—and I admit to having that "it's all over" feeling as we sorted through what to take and what to leave. What a damaging point of view for the elderly to hold. Must we cling to dusty old belongings in order to protect ourselves from what we are led to believe is our road to useless-ness? It can seem to us, and even to our families, that getting rid of our life's treasures signals our end and shuts the door on any confident thinking about a future. Not true. Not true.

I don't want to dwell on those days, but there was real pain in thinking that we were discarding belongings because this was the end of any meaning-ful life. Actually, once this difficult task was done, I found that it was instead the beginning of a new and different time—our elder years. (Oh, let us hope to have a few happy ones, please.)

My daughter and I decided that we would move before we sold the house, so we put red dots on all the furniture that we wanted to take and all the boxes of books and dishes that had to go with us. We cleaned out our closets and sent bags and bags of discarded clothes to Goodwill. The movers, recommended by our new home, were excellent and did their assigned duty quickly and easily. Planet X, here we come, just like that—fast and simple—after all the mental anguish. Our proposed new life had now become our reality.

Although seamless, the move was very tiring. We knew where each piece of furniture would go because we had mapped it out, and our children put things in closets and cabinets and hung all our pictures. Our things looked more at home than we did. We were moved. I can still see Dear Husband sitting on his beloved couch looking around with a little smile on his face. His smug, satis-fied look told me that in some way this seemed like home to him. He turned on his TV and settled in, and I think the fact that he had a freezer to hold his chocolate ice cream made it OK. Believe it or not, after all our worry and sub-terfuge, he seemed content. Me? I was exhausted, physically and emotionally. That first night was one of those nights when I could not sleep even though

I needed it so badly. I lay there itching and aching and wondering … what would the next day bring?

Several residents and one or two staff members welcomed us on moving day, and I very much needed the welcome. They would peek in the door and tell us that we would all get together later. What a hospitable thing to do, and something I try to imitate to this day. I recently spoke to another resident about this, and she, too, mentioned how much she appreciated those first welcomes from older tenants. Ironically, although we humans have a need to belong, when crashing a new group, we wonder if these are our people, or whether we will be happy with them. In a group of over one hundred new, old persons, I have discovered I have grown close to some, but not all. Isn't this as it always is?

I may have been welcomed, but I remember sitting on the edge of my bed that first night, looking out an unfamiliar window and thinking, what a dull view of nature. I must admit, even after all my positive talk, every optimistic thought I had deserted me, and I cried and cried. I cried out of exhaustion. I cried as I said a final goodbye to what had been and would never be again. Not ever. I don't think my family ever knew how much I hurt that first night.

After taking a couple of days to recoup, I began thinking about what to do with the stuff we left behind and how to sell the house. There were still some monumental tasks ahead, and I welcomed them because they gave me something to do. Daughter and I returned to what we had called home, and the visit gave me a big shock—not because I wanted to return, but because it hit me that what I was looking at was excess. I was viewing a now unlived-in house full of discarded antiques and junk, and lots of both. That so much was left after we had taken all we really needed made this residue seem like gross overindulgence, which, as I think about it, really is an American disease. This, more than anything that had happened, made me realize how far our lives are from those who live in much of the rest of the world. We middle-class Americans are indeed spoiled. We have too much stuff.

Even though we were all tired, we now had to get rid of this massive clutter. What to do? I called two antique dealers I respected and asked who they would recommend to conduct an estate sale. (It's a good idea to get a recommendation for such a sale.) Both named an antiques dealer, the owner of a beautiful shop, who also conducted estate sales. With this recommendation, I made an appointment with her.

Our meeting with L. was positive. She was a well-dressed, fortyish woman whom we immediately assessed as a take-charge person. Yes, I felt good about leaving the disposal of these things to her. For a percentage of the net sales, she would set up and conduct the sale, furnish the help needed, and clean out the entire house. Sold! The short contract we wrote stipulated that she would conduct a three-day sale, provide staff to see that items were not stolen, and ensure that everything left over after the sale would be taken out of the house and donated to Goodwill or other charities. That was important to me because I didn't want to be left with a load of stuff that hadn't sold.

I took one more look-see through the house, taking a few odd pieces I hadn't thought to take before, and then left the rest up to her. We had made a good choice. She immediately took charge, scooted us out of the house, pulled in her team of gofers, and went to work. The recommendations I had received from friends gave me peace that she was on the level; if you decide to dispose of possessions in this manner, be sure you ask for recommendations. Some of my friends have had things missing when they turned over their estate to the wrong dealer and were not as happy with the results. There are good and not so good estate-sale moguls. Be forewarned.

L. set aside three days to mark items and use her magic to make every-thing look desirable. I was so happy that she was taking the necessary time to get things priced and ready for the sale, and doubly pleased that she wanted me to go through everything to see if I agreed with her pricing. For the most part, we had no problem agreeing. However, I had to remember that I would never get top dollar for our stuff, and I admit that it hurt to see some precious pieces I paid a mighty dollar for priced at so much less. I told myself that unless I wanted to rent a shop and sell this hoard of stuff retail, piece by piece, I would never get full dollar. Again, I had to remind myself that it's just stuff.

I stayed far away from the actual sale. It's a bit severe to watch things you enjoyed living with leave the house they had called home, and at what we owners usually feel is a cheap price. It hurts. So for three days L. would call to report how the sale was going. Her advertising drew in large crowds of shop-pers, who were buying and buying. Everybody loves a bargain, and as a result we had a bit more money to put into the bank for future expenses. I began to feel that the past, which had been full of so many happy moments, but recently so many problems, was behind us and that maybe, just maybe, we could look forward to a calmer future, whatever that would be.

My daughter took over much of the contact work concerning the sale, and when I arrived at the house the day after, there were three neat piles of goods to be picked up by three different charities. It was a strange feeling to think that the furniture and things we had lived with for years were scattered all over the city and now belonged to people we didn't even know. I remember going to a local antique mall a few months later and seeing some of our things. I felt like grabbing them and saying, "Mine! Mine! These are mine!"

I found that the new friends we were meeting at Planet X had disposed of their stuff in several different ways. Some had had their kids take it all and do what they wanted with it, some had given much away to friends and sold some pieces individually, while others still had their homes and were going through the years of accumulation piece by piece. One couple took a year to sort through these memories. My advice, for what it's worth, is to spend only so much time on past stuff and look to a clutter-free future as soon as possible. Another caveat: children of aging parents, don't feel guilty because you don't want Mother's lace doilies. It's a different era and our stuff doesn't always fit with your stuff.

Before we knew it, all our clutter was now someone else's clutter. Wisely, after the mess of the move and the sale were over, we hired a recommended house cleaner to give the place a good scrubbing. When all of that was complete, our main task was to interview a few real estate agents. It is no easy task to find the right agent. The problem is compounded by the fact that we are more comfortable selling our home if we feel that our property is in good hands. One or two agents indicated that they were willing to represent both the buyer and the seller, but we were encouraged not to accept this, probably because in such a deal, how can the agent keep from having divided loyalties? We were lucky in that a neighbor of our daughter happened to be highly recommended to us, and she led us beautifully through all the ifs, ands, and buts of current real estate jargon. Believe me: get used to signing your name and reading between the lines. That was, to me, the hardest part of selling our home—all the detail work.

The list price she recommended succeeded in getting prospective buyers interested and brought in several bids. There are so many subtle factors present in real estate sales today. In our legalistic world, even though some sellers may be wise enough to act as their own agent, I personally would not dare to sell a house without a real estate sales professional unless I had the advice of a lawyer.

The average person is just not aware of all the little nuances and regulations strewn throughout a bill of sale.

If one were to tour our older home, he or she would see that work needed to be done. This meant we either fixed all the dingers, or we sold it as is—in other words, at a price that would make it clear that we knew the house needed work. This would later protect us when the prospective buyers wanted an inspection. The inspection would be made, but with the understanding that regardless of what was found, the price would not change. Our agent took pictures, and suddenly our home of forty-seven years was up for sale. We were fortunate because the population of the metro area was growing rapidly, causing a sellers' market at the time we sold.

Between the contract and the closing we had to contend with the inspection, the condition of the sewer, and never-ending questions from the prospective buyers. That is to be expected, and our real estate agent led us through all this. Is there mold? Radon? Carbon monoxide? Is the sewer broken? I had no idea if these hazards existed, so I suffered through each check of the premises, worried that one seemingly small problem might blow the whole deal. In this state there are certain restrictions. For instance, a bad sewer line must be fixed before a home is sold. Our agent can be applauded for looking out for our interests until the contract was signed and the money was in the bank. I can tell you that was a very good feeling.

Real estate has been a good investment for our generation. Many of us bought our home in the 1960s or 1970s at what now seems to be a ridiculous price, and today we are selling at a high enough price to allow us to afford the high rents common in senior residential communities. Many of the residents of our senior home are living here on the money from real estate investments or pensions earned in better days. The next generation will not meet such good times, I fear, and must look out for their financial welfare long before their senior years.

When I was teaching senior high school economics, I always advised students not to live from paycheck to paycheck. Save a little as you go along if you can. Today it is difficult for young people not to spend all they earn, but the habit can make one a wage slave and, most alarmingly, nothing is put aside for a rainy day or retirement.

So, now the house was sold and the stuff was gone. It had finally happened; we had disposed of our home and our clutter of forty-seven years, and more. The next day daughter called me and said, "I don't really know what this feeling is that I am having, but I feel funny." *I knew the feeling.* Suddenly, I felt homeless. Perhaps the word should be *rootless,* and the utmost question at that time was, how do I get over this? I didn't like the sensation; it didn't feel healthy at a time when it was so important for us to be able to view this move as a time to remake our lives and to create a more positive future for whatever time we had remaining.

I had no desire to wallow in nostalgia for a past I could not bring back. But grief, even for a home, needs its time in one's heart. Would it be too sentimental to take just a wee moment to let my lip quiver, and my eyes well up with tears out of respect for the place where we had raised our children, made our neighborhood friends, and lived for so many of our years? Goodbye, home. I won't miss having to paint your face or dress your insides or outsides, but, gee, I sure would like to live those years over once again. Goodbye, old home.

One year later I drove by our former home. There stood a snowman and a snowdog held by a leash, gracing what had been our front yard. They looked so at home there. With his tree twig arms, the snowman waved at us and blew us a kiss, and I felt the warmth of joy that another family was growing, loving, and living happily in our old home. Yes, the blackbirds continue to sing on the riverbank, and all is as it should be. Our life was not over; it had only changed location.

For us, it was time to look at our own future in this unknown new world. Would we be lucky enough to have much of a future? We did not know. We were now at an age at which we live one day at a time. We needed to be grateful for the days we've had and to look carefully at what we wanted our future to hold. We needed to attend particularly to this, the last part. Our culture may not look to these final years as important, and even we may not count them as significant, but contrary to contemporary thought, these last days can indeed be the most vital portion of our lives. I know the last three-plus years have proved powerfully rich for me. Goodbye, old home. I pray you will be well cared for as we move on to new friends, a new home, and a creative future without you.

Home is people. Not a place. If you go back there after the people are gone, then all you can see is what is not there any more.

—Robin Hobb, *Fool's Fate*

FIVE

A Society of Strangers

If you're brave enough to say goodbye, life will reward you with a new hello.
—PAULO COELHO, *THE ALCHEMIST*

And now we come to the part that would make a difference in our lives. Had we made the right decision? Rather, had *I* made the right decision? Had we arrived at a spot-on place to hang our Home Sweet Home sign? It wasn't going to be enough to simply have a dwelling, as far as I was concerned. I wanted a home. I wanted a place where I felt comfortable, where I could make friends, and where I could do things—things that would feed my needs. I hope someone from corporate senior care reads what I just wrote. I think everyone my age would agree with my words. We want a home.

I have talked to many fellow residents here at Planet X, and a lot of them end the conversation with, "… but it isn't home." Well, according to my dictionary home is "the place where one resides," but according to our heart, it is that place where we feel comfortably at ease; where the heart tells us, "Rest, relax. This is where you belong." Regardless of any heartfelt feelings we might have, we had arrived at a new address and we had hope. Always hope.

I will admit that it was easier to anticipate leaving our home and possessions than it was to do so. For the first few weeks in our new home I felt caught between goodbye and hello. My emotions waffled wildly from sad to happy, and I wavered from a sense of having found a home to an unexpected homesick reaction. I guess that was normal, wasn't it? Here I had thought I was ready to shed the problems inherent in an old house, and instead I was shedding a tear or two.

I have since talked to others who made this move, and some of us had similar reactions. Although I immediately experienced the exhilaration of seeing fresh faces and the enticement of new activities, I still yearned for my comfortable past life. At least in hindsight I recognized it as having been comfortable, while I felt a bit of stiffness and tentativeness in moving into our new home, which seemed to be such a public place.

My life's book had opened to a new page. I hadn't lived in such a common setting with others since college, and needless to say, that was a long time ago. I struggled with the doubt that the place my actions had brought us to was right, and I wrestled with this unhinged feeling of discovering myself in a place where I felt I didn't belong. Closing my eyes, I crossed my fingers and hoped I was wrong. Perhaps the good fairy would make it all right. Thank heavens for hope.

If you are considering such a move as ours, resign yourself to the fact that there is a big difference between single housing and communal living. This is not communal living of the kind we were familiar with in the sixties, when those who joined communes shared similar outlooks and beliefs. We have come to find that our new home is inhabited by an extremely homogeneous, yet diverse, group of persons. Sometimes the differences are subtle, and at first glance we might call ourselves "middle-class, virtually white older America." Few black families have so far broached the ramparts, although many of us are looking forward to that time, and I understand that Planet X now has an outreach program.

When we moved in, even though we were all seniors, some were almost old enough to be my mother, and I was eighty-two. The average age here is eighty-three. As the twenty-three-year-old grandson of a friend said, "I never saw so many old people in my life." (Slight pause here to say a word for closer relations between family members.)

Yes, here we are all old, but also diverse: right wing, left wing, no wing, various religious affiliations, on the prowl and contentedly single, ready to rumble and don't bother me. It's an impossible group in which to get a majority opinion. There is J., who goes to the gym almost every day, and K., who plays golf twice a week and is fairly fit and agile. There are those who must rely on their motorized scooter or electric wheelchair to even get to dinner. Some have very little physical disability, while others are crippled with Parkinson's or MS or some other ailment. High blood pressure, pacemakers, glaucoma, macular degeneration, and diabetes are our neighbors, and the walkers outside the dining room look like cars in a Walmart parking lot. Some minds are in quite good shape while others are trying hard. Accept the fact that in what is known as independent living, if there is an empty apartment to fill, almost any minor, or even major, illness will be overlooked, and there is a wider variety of health issues present than the management might want to admit. *Aging in place* is probably better terminology for what we have here.

Shortly after we arrived, a seventy-five-year-old woman who still played pickleball moved in. Her reaction was interesting. "This place makes me feel so old," she complained. "I wasn't prepared for all the old people." Had she looked in the mirror? Needless to say, this feeling of being old before her time prompted her to move out a few months later.

I, too, felt like I had been suddenly transported into an alien land. I, who loved to wear my PJs and slop around drinking my morning coffee, read our corporate directives and found that we weren't supposed to wear slippers outside of our apartment. And then, well-clad and -clothed, we found that around every corner was a someone to whom we must always give a toothsome smile. Always smile, with the hope that this is the universal signal that we are really OK to get to know.

The fact, however, was that I felt somewhat overwhelmed by being surrounded, almost simultaneously, by one hundred sixty or more new persons. Who could remember their names? Jim, Bill, Sarah, Joyce, Elaine, Ellen, Evelyn, Loretta, Lynette, Louisa? I knew I'd never remember them all. And remember last names? Only rarely. Everyone was a stranger, and I assumed they felt the same toward me.

Through my exhaustion and somewhat homesick haze, I woke up that first day glad that the move was over. But as I walked through the halls of our new home, this alien soil, it became a kind of no man's land to me. I hated the hallways; the colors were chosen to be warm and friendly, but to me they seemed dismal and harsh. Looking back, I wonder why I reacted this way. Perhaps the tightness and containment of these long, narrow passageways were a symbol of the trapped feeling I was experiencing. My chest felt tight, and all I could think was we, *I*, made a terrible mistake. How many times will I have to walk through these hallways and feel like this? I have to admit that even after three years, I still don't feel responsive to the halls. I think others may feel as I do, for almost everyone has decorated their doors and set little tables next to them with seasonal décor galore in an effort to give the place some warmth and softness.

I couldn't help wondering, at that first light, on my first morning, with the fatigue of the move still on my shoulders, if I would feel this way for the rest of my life. Oh, dear. There was only one thing to do, and that was to let time work its magic and make all my sad thoughts go away, and in the meantime to somehow get some control over myself and the situation. Once again, I needed to find my spunk.

To that end, I promised myself that I would give the place a chance. We have, since these early days, settled in nicely, and I have discovered that not everyone feels as I did. There are those who profess discontent with aspects of our new home for their remaining days here. Some move out, while others just complain. Yet one friend, on her first visit, walked in and said, "Wow. This is for me," and has been a happy camper ever since. I would say that most find more to like here than to dislike.

The building here at Planet X is large and sprawls up and down across a small hill, making it hard to find one's way around. I know it sounds strange, but you would have to see it to understand. The lobby ends up being on the second floor, for there is no first floor in the middle section of the building, and this is confusing to new residents. There are four floors of apartments, plus all-occasion rooms for games, exercise, therapy, and activities. It takes a while for it to feel like a cozy little home.

I made one very good move right away, and that was to walk the entire building, all four floors. This gave me a better idea of where everything was, and somehow this reassured me a bit. I began right away to put down very small roots. I reminded myself that the next step was to get used to all the humanity that lived here and to discover how I would fit into this strange new family. I say family because that is what it is; we are with each other so much of the time that after three years I can honestly say we are truly a part of this aging family, or we should be. Some are closer than others, of course, but given the chance, we do care. One leaves and we suffer a little bit, or even a lot. Each moment can bring good or bad news about our neighbors. At breakfast this morning I asked B. how his ninety-five-year-old wife was. (I had heard that she fell.) The news was not good. As happens too often with the elderly, A. had broken her hip with her fall and faced surgery. Not good news.

I began to think of Planet X as a city, with each hallway a street. I could now find my way around this new megalopolis, but I still didn't know those who lived within, and worst of all, I didn't feel like I lived here either. I recall lying in my bed the first few nights staring out the window and wishing I could see my old familiar sights as I gazed into the dark. Strange that I would miss such a small part of our past life. I missed the misshapen tree and the birds and squirrels that had played tag in its gnarled life. As I aged I had somehow identified with that old tree. I didn't miss my stuff, but I did miss that hoary old tree.

Just as I have heard others say, at first I was amazed at all the people I saw with their walkers and wheelchairs. I don't know why this is the reaction of so many of us, except that, like most Americans, we haven't yet agreed that we, too, deserved to be called "old." Associating with all these gray-haired souls made me feel like I had been relegated to a separate classification of life. For a while, I truly felt like I had been sent to live on a real Planet X: a planet of all white-haired aliens. Yes, these first few days were when I went from feeling mentally shelved to physically shelved.

It's impossible to describe anyone as gray-haired here. Everyone is gray-haired, or almost everyone. I'm not sure I'm expressing this in a way that readers will understand, but I suddenly felt that we were in a far-off world; this shelf I found myself on was deep and distant, a thousand mental miles from the active, doing world I had been used to before my husband's illness threw us into oblivion. Because of its separateness and my own feeling of strangeness, I decided to call our new home Planet X, a place beyond all reality. Instead of being a vigorous part of the adult world, we had suddenly entered a new, captive, unknown space, and I needed to find out what life was like in this outer interstellar world.

I soon learned that the dining hall is the center of everything: eating is very important here. It was obvious from the very beginning that the dining room is Zone A for socializing, complaining, and a lot of fun. Dining can take anywhere from one hour to two depending on the service, the conversation you're having, and how fast things are moving in the kitchen. Add to this the fact that mealtime is when we are all at our most visible. I well remember walking to that first meal and feeling like every eye was on us, and they were. Older residents here are always aware of new faces—not in a critical way, but curious about who is moving into the neighborhood. Yes, this is a neighborhood, and we learned very quickly that it is filled with a most varied and interesting group of people, contrary to the fact that they seem so akin. Did I say interesting? Yes, indeed. Here and in later chapters I will describe some of them for you. They are worth knowing.

At that first meal, as Husband and I stood there like deer in the headlights, dear L., who is still my good friend, motioned to us to come and sit with her and W. I was relieved. L. is one of those people who views no one as a stranger, and our friendship has thrived from that day forward. W. was the white-haired jester of the manor and we both enjoyed his happy attitude. W.

never grew up, and although wisdom was hidden beneath the clown visage he adopted, there was little doubt that he was living life his way. In his lifetime he had traveled to many of the world's exotic places, and he filled his space with smiles and positive vibes. W. looked a lot like Santa, and one year at Christmas he wheeled his chair to all the ladies' tables asking, "Do you want a kiss?" And he would give the diner a chocolate kiss. Not funny? Not cute? Come on! Who could not like a guy like this? However, diabetes had done serious damage to W.'s foot, and as a result he needed that motorized chair.

I had met W. earlier, while we were moving in. Some of his first words to me were, "I came here to live, not to die." I have treasured that wise message ever since. A good man with a strong thought, and I have tried to hold on to that vision. Although three years later my friend, my jolly white-haired, white-bearded, dear friend is now gone, he will always be in my heart.

Needless to say, we gladly sat with W. and L. and enjoyed a wonderful brunch. It made us feel almost at home. Almost. Lesson one in a senior home: Don't wait for tomorrow to be friends. Carpe diem is the motto, for who knows what tomorrow will bring.

There were a few of those early meals that weren't as pleasant as this first one. It is so embarrassing to ask someone if you may join them at their table only to be told, kindly but firmly, that the seats are taken. I was unaware that there is a terrific territorial quality to mealtime among select residents, and it took a bit of getting used to. This is each person's home, and there are certain souls with whom some of them are used to sharing a table. They have grown comfortable with said dinner partners, and now that I have been here longer, I understand that better. Now I see it through a wider lens and know that it is not necessarily dismissive, but a sign of needing security. However, when we were new, it wasn't a pleasant welcome. Some residents have sat at the same table with the same people for two to three years, but there are others who enjoy dining and becoming acquainted with a wider assortment of friends. Just as in the real world individual quirks have to be accepted and tolerated, the same is true here. As I said, this is a very diverse group of people.

Some of us asked to be seated at a table of six or eight. With this number we found that we not only had more fun, but we got to know more people. Dinner partners came and went, and we always enjoyed our mealtime. Planet X has since decided to dictate where we will sit, and we wait to be seated by a "hostess." C'est la vie.

From the very first, living with so many dissimilar others took some adjustment on my part. Some residents seemed so inward that it was as though they were barely there. I can think of one lady I've seen three times in two years. Some have their meals delivered so they don't have to come to the dining room, and others come and pick up meals, then scurry back to eat alone. In the three years we have been here I have seen one woman come to dinner only two times, while others show up for every meal, seeming to want to know everyone, and have no trouble conversing and projecting self-confidence by the barrel. If I had not recognized differences in personalities before, I certainly have since moving to Planet X.

We began to discover that, yes, this was even more like a college dorm than we had imagined, with the exception that much longer lifetime behaviors also complicate the picture. Yes, we elders have all developed favorite quirks over the course of our lives. Some of us wonder why everyone doesn't "do as I do" and "think as I think." If one has done something the same way or eaten the same foods for seventy or eighty years, it begins to seem like the only way it should be done, which accounts for some of the complaining we hear about meals and service. The food is the first thing carped about in most senior homes. I think there are reasons for this; in the first place, food assumes an importance in the elder day, and as I've said, we've become accustomed to having it the way we like it. I wouldn't be the head chef here for any amount of money. We have Chef's Chat, which we will discuss later, but it is an exercise in futility to try to please both the hot salsa and the mild salsa residents.

I must admit, at first I was unduly critical of residents and their habits. I found it odd to see them rush to dinner and then rush back to their apartments to watch *Jeopardy*. Along the way we should have learned that there are all kinds of persons in this world. And now, in our more limited world, and after a lifetime of learning, we should be able to handle the diversity. But that is not always the case. As a warning, I will introduce you to what Joan Chittister says in her book *The Gift of Years*. Read this and you will approach the shelf with caution:

> The truth is that older people tend to come in two flavors—the sour ones and the serene ones. The sour ones are angry at the world for dismissing them from the rank and file of those who run it and control it and own it and are not old in it. They demand that the rest of the world seek them

out, pity them, take their orders, stay captive to their scowls. The serene ones live with soft smiles on their aging faces, a welcome sign to the world of what it means to grow old gracefully.[1]

The more I read this quote, the less I agree with it. I agree that it isn't pleasant to be summarily dismissed from the ranks of the movers and shakers of the world, but I really don't see elders as wanting to be pitied, nor do most of those I know want anyone to be captive to their moods. I'm afraid Chittister is a victim of our social mindset, seeing the elderly as they are seen by a large percentage of our society. I suggest she look deeper.

In the last two years I have met both kinds of elders, those who appear sweet and those who appear a bit sour, and yet I assure you that the majority of these who are our neighbors are definitely of the more serene variety. If I have any criticism it is that perhaps they are too apt to be serene and are not willing to fight city hall now and then. It is too easy to let things slide because we feel too tired or old to make the effort. It is too easy to say, "Oh, well," rather than tussle with the corporation for a needed addition to our home or our daily life. Rather than classify our generation as Chittister does, consider one's own reaction to the bitter and the better. Three years of living with such a diverse group of people has taught me to focus on my own attitudes. It is enough to try to avoid the sour in my own soul. Often illness, loneliness, or other problems cause that scowl on an elderly face.

Actually, I find it is difficult to diagnose the cause of the mood swings I encounter around here. Living communally has, however, opened my mind and heart a bit to realize that we never know what pain lies in someone's path that may have severely affected them, so it's best to say, rather positively, "I've met a lot of friends and good-hearted people. Some are even nicer than I am."

I know for the first few weeks I was guilty of falling into that negative trap of pity for myself and criticism of others. It's an easy yoke to don: first, if we label someone as an old grump, it relieves us from having to look deeper, and it becomes a quick method of choosing non-friends. We can superficially and quickly divide a group into the goodies and the baddies. However, the question is, do we sometimes miss a real gem of a person when we judge others so quickly? I know I have.

But I have grown, and now I try to listen to that still, small voice in my head that says to me now and then, "Try to understand." For I ask myself, at the final accounting, will the sometimes bitter person lose more points with the Creator, or will I be the loser, if I am the one who waxes judgmental toward him or her?

I have come to believe that complaining, or what I like to call "voicing a suggestion," is often needed when we want to change things that need changing, but judging another is quite another thing. Funny I should recall it this late in my life, but I remember that my mother always told me that God had a big black book, and every time we did something wrong he wrote our name in it. I smile when I think of how that book has influenced my life, and still does, at least subconsciously.

Looking back, I know I was as much at fault as anyone for my early negative reaction to both the place and its people. I'm sure my name went into that black book numerous times for the negative thoughts I had. But I learned, slowly. One day while looking at the schedule I noticed they had exercise classes on Tuesdays and Thursdays. I decided to try a class, and as I entered, I saw that they were doing exercises sitting down. Oh, no, I thought. Exercising in chairs? I'm not that old. I guess this is how it is with old people. (I still had not accepted myself as being old.) However, as the charming young woman began the class and we started to exercise, I changed my mind. Chair exercises can be quite tiring, but also very good for stretching the muscles. She also found a way to give us some good aerobic exercise, and chair or no chair, I felt much better after the half hour of making my body work. My prejudice was exposed. This class that had seemed to be for old people, and something I turned up my nose at, proved to be just what both Husband and I needed.

One of the things I have enjoyed the most here at Planet X is taking our little dog, Lucy, outside several times a day. According to the rules, I have to keep her on a leash, and I was afraid she would feel confined here compared to her life in the big backyard she had left behind. However, Lucy really is not an outdoor dog, and her favorite pleasure has turned out to be running to everyone she meets and giving them a kiss. Lucy loves everyone, and loves attention. As a result, almost everyone in our new home adores her and she thoroughly enjoys everyone. Well, not everyone. There are a few animal haters here, or maybe they are just dislikers who are upset by pet messes and averse to seeing dogs in the lobby. Living with others makes us aware that there are those who have a serious fear of dogs, or who are allergic. Planet X is listed as a pet-friendly place, but attention must be paid to those who are not pet friendly. That, again, is part of communal living.

Compromise, however, is the most needed and least practiced commodity around here. It is beginning to sink in: this is what shared living is all about, and I do believe it is in this arena that positive change in senior care will occur in the future. The winds of decision don't always blow one's way, and some folks here understand compromise while others do not. Even the corporate owners have trouble with compromise. Perhaps I should say *especially* the corporate owners. Patience and tolerance and thinking inclusively and creatively are often the answer, but not always available. There is often not the kind of management that sees the advantage in putting something in place with the least disruption, or trying to find a compromise between Corporate and residents. Yet, to my way of thinking, this would be real management.

When one is sold on living in an apartment in such a place as Planet X, one (I) expects to receive what is promised as understood in the contractual agreement. Right? Well, corporate ownership dictates that there are always many voices speaking and decoding, or not decoding. Communication regarding the yeses and nos and the cans and can'ts and the wills and won'ts can be quite slippery. One staff member indicates that *this* is corporate policy and another says it is *that*. This happened to us. We were told that the convenient laundry room about twenty steps from our new apartment was where we could do our washing. This was a factor in choosing our apartment. (We do our personal laundry, although Housekeeping does our sheets and towels.) A few days after we moved in, the basket was full and I waddled it down to the assigned laundry, which was two doors away. Sorry, I was told; this laundry was only for Maintenance's use. The staff had taken it over to launder those sheets and towels for us. Where was I to go? Where were thirty to forty other third floor residents to go? The staff pointed to the first floor and more or less said, "It's all yours." I didn't really mind going that far to clean the duds, but I was bothered that I'd been told something before moving in that had proved false.

I sent a grievance to the executive director, who came and chatted about my grumble. Her answer: "I'll look into it." Well, that was three years ago, and we are on her fourth replacement as executive director, and I'm still doing the duds on the first floor. Rule #1: If you really want a guarantee, get a definitive answer in writing. And if you put in a request to have something done, keep checking on it. Some things at Planet X take months to get accomplished, and I've learned that in senior living some things never arrive. They may always be just thinking about it, and putting things off is sometimes just a way to say no to a request. Is that management? Yes, I guess it can be called that.

This brings up another thing you can expect in senior residences: the director and the staff influence much of the attitude and atmosphere of the place. In three-plus years we have had four directors and will be starting on our fifth next month. Each has created his or her own ambience. Our first leaned toward "thinking about it" when approached about a change, leaving us at a loss to solve many problems. But the next director was good about giving us a straight-out answer. We might not like the answer, but at least we didn't feel that we were being led on. The third director was here one month then was promoted, and the fourth was here a few months but is now looking forward to semi-retirement. Number five is on his or her way and we will have to wait and see what lies in store for us.

Senior residences are like any other institution: they have rules to follow, but the director and staff provide the interpretation of the rules. I mentioned this once before, but it bears repeating: flexibility is present, but it is often hidden within the rules, which are many times cited when the occasion merits, and sometimes ignored when it doesn't. Hopefully the residences of tomorrow will understand the importance of allowing those who live here and pay the bills to have more of a voice in the day-to-day operations. What could it hurt? Giving up a little power, perhaps?

Now let me tell you about happy hour. Friday nights before dinner, wine, alcohol, and soft drinks are on tap with old-time music for all in the lobby. This is a great time for some, and alcohol seems to bring out more residents than almost any other enticement in the house. But watching elderly women balance martinis and manhattans on walker seats was a shocker the first time. It wasn't the beverages that bothered me, but that was a sight I had to get used to. Another thing was that everyone seemed to sit in little clutches, or little groups, that never seemed to say, "Come sit with us." W. was the only one who invited us to join him and his guests. At that time I was newbie shy and hesitant to break into what I saw as cliques. Friendliness has two sides, and that is something I had to remind myself of. I know most of the residents now and don't see them as hostile, and I have decided that my hesitancy about happy hour was my problem, not theirs.

Gradually we began to get acquainted, and as we got to know others' backgrounds, we found that there were often reasons for some residents to be a bit distant. There is a lot of pain in many of the backgrounds that residents may not want to discuss. I was getting some popcorn downstairs in the lobby one afternoon when a small, gray-haired, impeccably dressed lady came by. We began chatting, and I found out that she had lost two daughters and a husband.

This is a home for many widows and widowers, and it has been a greater change for them than for Husband and me. Age brings with it experiences, some of which leave an ache in the heart and can affect one's outer visage.

Tonight, while waiting for the dining room to open, a fellow resident and I began talking about our feelings about our first months at Planet X. She is a widow, and when I asked about her feelings she said, "I don't know if you would want to print them." Then she proceeded to tell me that she had had almost no say in moving here. Apparently her family, including her brother, had decided what she was supposed to do. She is still angry about it and looked at me with this expression of hurt, saying, "What business was it of his? I still don't feel like this is my home." Family members, be careful and considerate if you are involved in a major change regarding the life of a loved one.

As I began to get acquainted with others, I was surprised that I heard so many voice the sad view that almost everything was over for them. Life was done. I sensed that deep down they felt that they were just waiting out the time until the end. However, as I have said, there are just as many who play or party or volunteer and are ready to go and do at the drop of a hat. The more I see of elders' dispositions, the more I see, rather than Chittister's sour versus serene choice of mood, a choice expressed between depressed and lonely versus determined.

For me this has been one of the most difficult adjustments of my life, but I am enormously glad that we made the move. At first I really needed to talk to others and compare notes about our experiences. I didn't like to think of what I was feeling as homesickness, when I had made such a show of being forward looking and boasting about how happy I was to leave that old house behind. But the truth was, I needed to take some time to grieve the past and acclimate myself to a new future. Taking a bit of time to grieve is never time wasted, unless it extends into time forward.

Dear Husband, however, amazed us all and adjusted even more readily than I. We were all surprised that within a week he was in love with the place and chatting with one and all at meals. I could see how good it was for him to be here. All of his ill feelings about moving were forgotten. In this case the dementia did him a favor. At mealtime he shared war stories and jokes with others and really seemed to enjoy himself. He looked forward to going to all the meals and was the sweetheart of the group. The servers and residents still seem to enjoy his humor, kidding him about his love of chocolate ice cream. For the moment, his dementia is left behind.

He may not remember what he is going to do after dinner, or how to get to the lobby, but he can still think of jokes to make everyone laugh. It seems that the dementia has loosened his tongue and added to his sense of humor. Such a blessing. Some dementia patients aren't so lucky, but so far we haven't seen anything from him but a sweet, forgetful smile. My dear soulmate is simply a happy, aging old man with a bit of fun left in him. I can live with that. Occasionally, if taken out of his usual routine, he can act nervous and even erratic, so we watch and we wait, knowing that the time may come when he will need more structure than Planet X can provide. At present the two of us can manage reasonably well, but I worry when I see him having trouble negotiating steps, and I notice the shake that is developing in his hands.

When I saw his response to our new home, I knew we had made the right move. This move was just what he needed. Instead of crawling into a deeper hole, or spending every day without friends, he came into daily contact with more people, and the benefit of that has been immeasurable. Research has shown that this is good for all of us as we age.[2] However, even though he likes going to meals, he still prefers to spend part of his days between meals glued to his favorite couch, watching TV.

I'm so glad I resisted placing him in memory care and decided to move with him to our new home. We are still together, thank goodness, and we have both blossomed here, I a bit slower than he. Important to note, however: independent living is good for him because of his personality, and because I am here to call many of the shots. I would not consider independent living for a demented person living alone. We have had several move into and then out of Planet X. Dementia is not a stranger in most senior homes, but the confusion it causes can be extremely unsafe for a single demented person, particularly in the first months of getting acquainted with a new home. As an example of the confusion dementia can cause to the single resident, I recall our neighbor who could not remember where he was born. I discovered him one evening in a frightening position. He had entered an elevator but had not pushed the button. Apparently he had stood there in the silence, and he would have been there until someone else called for the elevator if I had not opened the door and seen him standing there. It scared me to death. In other incidents he was found wandering around the building and no one was sure he could find his way back to his apartment.

I can't explain why I had an initial downbeat reaction to life here, but even though I'm now an unfinished advocate of life here at Planet X, I had the harder adjustment. I had been positive all through the move, but once here I had the feeling that society was saying, "There's no longer any job you are capable of," placing me on the edge of uselessness—the shelf. Until I took a bit of time to think things out and study this change we were experiencing, I could only see the negatives.

These unwanted feelings of uselessness convinced me that I needed to look deeper into this thing that was happening to us called aging. Did I have anything to look forward to in elderhood? Was there going to be a future, or should I just give up and get in bed? Something was wrong with this. I felt that I had the rest of my life, whatever time that was, and I needed to know more about what this slice of life was like and how I could enjoy these years. Is there some reason I'm still around while others I grew up with are long gone? Is there something I need to accomplish? Something I have left undone? I don't know, but even though a walker may be a part of my later life, I don't want it to dominate my personhood. Dr. Spock was there for babies, umpteen books were written about "those difficult teen years," and Oprah, Dr. Oz, and Dr. Phil held the adult audience in their hands, so I began to try to find out who were the gurus for the aged generation. As I studied, I was shocked to learn that recent research looks at aging in a far more positive way than we sense from the general public. Aging is a process that begins at birth, and it is not a frozen, immovable tragedy. It is not an illness, and, believe it or not, our later years can be a satisfying time of life. Our generation is lucky to have senior care that has progressed a great deal since my mother's day. And now I have begun to envision what a perfect senior home would be like. I hope it will be ready for the boomers.

There is a fountain of youth: it is your mind, your talents, the creativity you bring to your life and the lives of people you love. When you learn to tap this source, you will truly have defeated age.

—Sophia Loren

SIX

There Is Life after Sixty-Five, for God's Sake!

Life is never made unbearable by circumstances, but only by lack of meaning and purpose.

—Viktor Frankl, *Man's Search for Meaning*

Viktor Frankl, whose wisdom came from painful years at Auschwitz, tells us that meaning, not happiness or success, is the driving force of human life: "When we are no longer able to change a situation, we are challenged to change ourselves."[1] Well, I certainly cannot change the fact that I am old. The next question comes naturally: is it possible to find this thing called meaning in this final thrust at life? With some elderly persons, it all seems to be a natural part of their lives, while others appear to be the victims of society's uncomplimentary view that old people are useless and inadequate. Welcome to the harmful image of elders in America that our culture has created for too many friends of mine. Please, America, listen! There is life after sixty-five, for God's sake.

No. We don't like to talk about aging or death, and we really don't even like to look in the mirror, so, my question is, is it possible to get us to look at the facts instead of the ideas we have simply assumed to be true concerning this phase of our life? The research I did about this time in my life has proved to be what is commonly known as an eye-opener. It has so helped me to personally find meaning in these latter years. And without a doubt, what I have learned has been tremendously helpful to me in caring for and understanding Husband. I didn't know I would be able to do this.

At eighty-five, I have my own medical problems, but, Friend, life is still good. I wake in the morning, ready to find another project or maybe just neaten up the apartment, and even though I have my moments, I am so glad that I have taken the time to learn more about this stage of life that now has me captive. Why? Of course part of my current good health I can attribute to luck, regular appointments with my doctor, and several necessary pills, but also my days have been made more pleasant because I have done due research about my old age. This has provided me with ways to value my age more positively than, I'm sad to say, my culture has.

I no longer accept the common societal view of people at eighty-five. Yes, I am still occasionally left out of younger persons' conversations, and I'm probably overlooked now and then, but I know what I think and who I am. There is life after sixty-five!

Obviously we are in a phase of life not held in high regard by our society, but, and this may be a surprise to you, Dear Reader, we oldsters can often blame ourselves for at least part of our problem. Keeping current with what is happening globally, locally, and within ourselves is something we elders sometimes ease out of when we get a bit tired and want to take it slow and easy. Do so, if that is mandatory for you and your health. But think again: what connections, and even how many years, are we willing to give up if we choose to mentally fade into the sunset?

Fade if you will, but my life's book will remain open only a short while—this is how we are all designed—and if there are attitudes and relationships and particulars that can possibly enrich this time, it would be a mistake for me not to educate myself to those possibilities.

When I arrived at the magic age of sixty-five, contrary to what my culture might say about it, I didn't feel useless. As a matter of fact I felt little different than I had at forty-five. I recognized that old age was beginning to attack those in my age bracket, but I had to wonder: what is my life supposed to be at this age? To answer that question for myself, I used the tools I had close at hand—my library and my computer—and began to do some diligent study regarding this thing called aging. I wanted to know facts, not just opinion or convention. What I came away with was a much needed education that significantly changed my thinking about my next few years.

The time spent was important to me in other ways as well. It helped me know more about what I should or could expect from those who were presenting themselves to me as caregivers of older Americans. I believe my most important lesson was realizing the extent to which contemporary research results differ from the collective public view of what to expect when we're old.

It is no secret that, unlike many other cultures, Americans see old age as dismal, depressing, and gloomy; it too often dooms elders to the shelf—and from there to the grave. How did we arrive at this sad attitude? How did we get this way?

Believe it or not, there were times in our past that elders were treated with respect. Powdered wigs were worn sometimes for medical reasons, but younger people seem to have affected this habit to make themselves look older, and, therefore, perhaps able to garner more respect. The proper conduct among the young was to obey their elders, and view them with awe probably more than affection. (There was, even then, an emotional distance between young and old.) All of this began to change, say the historians, during the Revolutionary period. Just as the hippie years were a revolt of sorts against the establishment, the American Revolution was a time of early negative reactions against old age itself. Clothing styles began to change, designed to make one appear younger, and that trend has continued to this day.[2]

Over the years, terms of disrespect for the elderly came into use: gaffer, old fogy, old goat, fuddy-duddy, geezer, galoot, baldy, and some were tinged with a drop of cruelty, like old bag or old bat. Along with loss of respect, a family's responsibility for their aged began to break down, and old folks' homes and poorhouses came into being. To escape or put off falling into this senior quicksand, people began to lie about their age, and such sayings as "over the hill" and "one foot in the grave" became popular, indicating the ugliness of aging. Jack Benny and his "I'm thirty-nine" comment was well understood by America, usually followed by a humorous chuckle.

In 1937, sixty-five became the age at which one could earn full retirement benefits. This was changed in 1987 to gradually increase the age to sixty-six and finally to sixty-seven after several years. These ages came to be considered the arbitrary age(s) at which people were considered to be of lesser value in the workplace. We can grant that some persons need to retire at sixty-five, sixty-six, or sixty-seven, but others are active until much later. I wonder if most Americans are aware of how mandatory retirement policies have meant poverty for many older citizens who are still capable of a day's work. Today this prejudice is happening at even younger ages. Ask employment agencies how many jobs they have for anyone over forty-five. The euphemism for "you're too old" is "you're overqualified" (the use of which protects employers against violating the Age Discrimination in Employment Act).

The period after World War II saw great mobility in America, which led to the breakup of multigenerational families. Families often moved to homes in the suburbs, and Grandma was no longer seen as a useful member of a family team, but rather as a drain on its resources. Youth was on one side of life, and old age appeared as beyond any real life. The idea that old people could actually fall in love or have sex was, and is, embarrassing to many Americans (but I'm told the boomers have a different idea about this stereotype).

Along with the negative view of our age comes a denial of aging from those who are doing the aging: "You're only as old as you feel," "I'm sixty years young," "Sixty is the new forty." No matter how we deny we are old, the marketplace sees it differently, reminding us that old knowledge is outmoded. We are has-beens, and our thinking has become stuffy, passé, yesterday. This attitude has grown through the years into what is known today as a cult of youth. The fear of aging has taken many forms, and even we, the elderly, believe we are of little value. New fads and changing styles have taken the place of respect for the past, except on Memorial Day or Veterans Day.

In a recent program here at Planet X, a lip-synch act was introduced to us as "giving us a taste of what is happening in the real world." *Real world.* This comment was made by someone who works with elders every day, and made without a hint of realization that this introduction was a terrific downer for the audience.

Come to Planet X and live with us as we lose our friends and try to convince ourselves of our worth. This will give you a taste of the real world, or at least a taste of real life. Of course we old fogies are too out of touch to know what is happening in the real world. Although the junior staff in our particular old folks' home, such as the housekeepers, maintenance persons, and servers in the dining room, are friendly and seem to accept us as human, and the upper management is pleasant and capable, the final corporate voice often speaks to those who carry out their desires in a manner that does *to* the elder resident instead of working *with* them. Therefore, I question whether they see us as being capable of making decisions about our daily lives.

I am speaking in general here, and I shouldn't do that. There are staff members at all levels who get the message. We have a program director who asks via a survey every year what activities sound interesting to us, who we want to hear speak, and where we want to go. In most cases, however, rules are changed and added without considering the wishes of those who live here—we are expected to simply accept our world as it changes in corporate directions. Management becomes arbitrary rather than giving much attention to the needs or suggestions of those who live here.

It is easy, if one doesn't challenge it, to feel like an old geezer. It is all around us. A few nights ago we went to our favorite Chinese restaurant and had a luscious meal. On the way out, a fortyish lady said to her date, "Hey, hold the door for those old people." I guess she just had to add the "old," bless her heart. It was just a small thing, but *old* was an unnecessary adjective.

However, today a large portion of our once youthful population is growing older, and it's interesting that the baby boomers, who find they are getting much closer to the fuddy-duddy stage, are waking to the need for more research and money to be spent on the elderly. If you don't believe how much more interest is shown in old age now that we have seventy million boomers facing this downturn, search the internet for research on aging: research studies and articles abound. I will only mention a few studies here that I discovered, but I encourage you to use that new-fangled gadget, the computer, to check out the research for yourself. It has been one of the most hopeful things I have done for myself.

According to the research, we may be old but we still have meaning, we still sometimes make sense, and we can still help ourselves make life richer and healthier than it may be at present. The good news is that, because we don't like feeling insignificant, some of us are passionately motivated to fill this period of our lives with a wealth of living that has value and worth, instead of giving in to the passive role society has assigned.

I know, however, that I am not speaking for all in my generation. Some elders are happy to be done with involvement and want someone to think for them. As one friend said at lunch, "They're management. Let them manage." I'm just not one of these. And I have many friends who agree with me. In fact, I think I'm in the majority, and I hope some of the following research will show you what convinced me to want to keep some control over my life.

A report that lends professional weight to what our society thinks of elders in the twenty-first century is *Gauging Aging: Mapping the Gaps between Expert and Public Understandings of Aging in America.*[3] Created in 2015 by the Frameworks Institute (a coalition of eight of our nation's leading aging-focused organizations), this report maps the gap in the public view of older adults versus what the experts are saying about our age group.

According to the report, the public view places seniors in an "other" group to which they, the adults, do not belong. Being an other really relegates us, doesn't it? Younger people are the doers and we ... well, you name it. It sure sounds like we are the outsiders, or the *others*. One clue to the present public disinterest in old people is the fact that less has been spent on aging research than on many other areas of concern. This lack of cash has caused some of the most talented researchers to not go into the field. I sense that this information is saying to us: Why bother? They're just going to die, so forget it. We need to wake up to the fact that those who are young will not stay young forever and that what is learned about aging today will help us now and will help tomorrow's aging.

One Frameworks coalition member, the American Federation for Aging Research (AFAR), spells it out: "What if there was a condition that affected over 40 million people and no one noticed? There is. It's called Aging."[4] AFAR also says that, according to *Gauging Aging,* public perceptions of aging describe the process as:

1. *Someone else's problem.* They see the aged as an "otherized" group to which they do not belong.
2. *Undesirable* and associated with decline and deterioration.
3. *Inevitable.* They fail to see the years of life which we still may have left, and only see us through a fog of inevitable loss.
4. *Isolated.* A majority of the public perceives elders only as a personal or family problem. We become a duty for family rather than something the public should be concerned with. Yet, ironically, fewer elders are living with children than ever before.
5. *Fatalistic.* Society seldom sees any good coming from aging, nor does it see any reason to research what support or policies could help this segment of the population. "They'll just die anyway." *(They?)*
6. *Out of sight and out of mind.* "If we don't see them, they're not here" is apparently what our society believes. Fear and misperception ultimately fuel a lack of attention for older adult health. Keeping the problems of elders under wraps does little to remedy impediments to health as the total group grows older, and this lack of attention causes a continual, accumulative need that is unaddressed.[5]

As I write, lawmakers are considering cutting Medicaid and Medicare monies for expensive treatments. It is an ongoing struggle to keep the benefits earned in recent years.

More dollars devoted to research today would mean better care for our younger members as society ages. But this is long-term thinking, and we Americans are not so good at that. Many great suggestions to improve our lives have been proposed since I've lived at Planet X, but they sometimes get caught in the corporate budget. The need for new exercise equipment to replace outdated equipment has been ignored, and resident requests for better nutrition and more attention paid to vegetarians and those with allergies are met with comments that this is independent living and the corporation doesn't cater to such needs—this said when Corporate is currently touting the concept aging in place. Aging in place is the drawing card to keep apartments full, but it is called independent living when one wishes to save corporate funds.

Another interesting theory was initiated by psychologist Erik Erikson and his wife, Joan. They advanced a theory of human development that initially included eight stages from infancy to old age, with wisdom as the focus of the eighth stage. The pair created the stages as they were experiencing them themselves, and after Erik's death in 1994, Joan added a ninth stage of very old age. She believed that "aging is a process of becoming free" and should not be treated as the opposite.[6]

Daniel Goleman, a well-known writer and psychologist who in the 1980s interviewed the Eriksons, sums up their work thusly: "They depict an old age in which one has enough conviction in one's own completeness to ward off the despair that gradual physical disintegration can too easily bring."[7] This sounds a bit like Viktor Frankl's exhortation to find meaning. The Eriksons urged people in their eighties and nineties to set goals that match their capabilities and personality.

One important suggested way for elders to ward off despair, find meaning, and strengthen wisdom is to attend classes in guided autobiography, or a life's review.[8] We also call this creating a memoir. The Eriksons' eighth and ninth stages are a time when we look back and evaluate the success or lack of success we've had in life. Depression and a feeling of failure or lack of accomplishment can lead to an old age of bitter misery. Rather than succumb to such a feeling, the research I've seen suggests that we need to look at this later age as a second chance, a chance to leave a happier legacy, if it seems necessary, or to look back with a more positive slant on our lives, feeling that we have grown and outlived some of our faults. The goal, of course, is to find some final sense of completion before our magic book of life closes.

This is a worthy message for our generation. Most of us born between 1925 and 1945 were shaped by the Depression, World War II, and later the Cold War and Korea. We were weaned on slow dancing or the jitterbug, and we now allow ourselves on the floor to dance when "geezer" music is played. The late David Halberstam, American journalist and historian, and a member of our generation, wrote in *Harvard Magazine* in 2005 that our generation is the "modest generation." It has often been called the "silent generation," but he believed that to be a misnomer. Instead, he called us the Frank Sinatra generation. As he said, that is our comfort level. Raised on the radio, we are a half-step behind the speed of news and change shown on TV. Fads, a love of fast action, and a faster-than-we-think change of affairs unsettle us, nor are we seen as an optimistic, outgoing generation, which can be a detriment to our maintaining a positive view of our old age.

Most of us don't want to cause a ruckus, but we are used to service from those from whom we purchase life's necessities. And although we may be quiet about it, we resent attitudes that allow social caregivers to more or less tell us what to believe and how to act. We are, according to Halberstam, "serious, somber, and reasonably skeptical."[9] We have a layer of restraint laid on by the cultural habits of our age and are reluctant to allow ourselves to display our feelings. Some of us have been hurt too often, and perhaps we have been told that others don't want to hear our pains—that they have pains of their own.

I have to add to this my personal concern that we are often afraid to venture too far out of our comfort zone to make contact with others. In his obituary of David Halberstam, journalist George Packer writes: "His colleague and friend Neil Sheehan … wrote, 'His insecurity showed … in his compulsion to be recognized and in his need to test himself.'"[10] Halberstam was a man of his generation. A man of our generation.

Regardless of our generational attitudes, what control do we have over our own aging? In his book *The Art of Aging: A Doctor's Prescription for Well-Being,* Dr. Sherwin Nuland acknowledges that we all age at different rates, but he points to newer evidence that shows that we can influence our own aging. Encouraging are the studies that show that the frequency of Alzheimer's is less in people who have pursued an active intellectual life. It's called being interested. It's called being alert to what is going on and caring. Intellectual stimulation can take many paths: avid reading and participation in a reading group, following politics, and taking a course with an academic theme are only some of the ways we can stimulate the mind. I have personally found the writing of *Shelved* to be a stimulant that I hope will keep me from mentally fading away too quickly. At eighty-five I still do not feel useless or close to having dementia. I am lucky.

Although my journey may not be your journey, we learn from one another. Let us read our newspaper, write letters to the editor, and complain about the food. Be heard and expect more from ourselves and from life. Read a good book and join a group or two. If we concentrate on living instead of preparing to die, it appears we have a lot to gain. We might even be able to keep some control over our life and our mind.

It is true that the mind is not the same at seventy as it was at twenty. In *The Art of Aging,* Dr. Nuland quotes Sir Francis Bacon: "Young men are fitter to invent than to judge, fitter for execution than for counsel, and fitter for new projects than for settled business."[11] Of course we must be aware of our present status. We are not as intellectually or physically quick as we once were, our reaction times are slower, and to differing degrees we can suffer from memory problems. We will not stay well forever, but in some instances our attitude toward our present life can keep us healthy and happy for more years than we probably deserve. Intellectual stimulation, cardiovascular exercise, and a healthy diet are a few of the tools that will help us interact meaningfully with our environment, allowing us to nurture the talents that experience and age provide. These talents are not negligible but may not be as visible as those of the doing generation—our younger adults.

Yesterday when I mentioned my book to a fellow elder, stressing that even at our age we can still do useful work toward our mind's desires, her cautious answer was, "Yes, but that's only true if you have good health. It's not true for those with illnesses." I disagree. I know her answer seems so true, and I'm sure it is true in certain instances, but haven't we, in our long lives, learned that appearances can be wrong? I have known so many my age who have had this or that sundry illness and have used their humor and their mind to look beyond the pain as much as they could—beyond the pain to a better mindset and ideas that take them away from their troubles. So much of our life depends upon attitude, and a happy mood can often help us transcend many of the problems and trying times brought on by declining health. Many of our friends here at Planet X have serious health issues: diabetes, the inability to walk unattended, blood clotting issues, decreased vision, pacemakers, chronic illnesses, and on and on. Nevertheless, I can assure you that we can continue to love life and stay actively involved in ventures and in the concerns of the day.

We are led to believe that pulling inward is the unswerving path of old age. Not so according to the *WebMD* article "The Secrets of Aging Well." This article describes one of the most unusual and widespread research studies ever conducted. It was called the Harvard Study of Adult Development and it studied more than eight hundred men and women starting in the 1930s. The study began with 268 Harvard undergrads, two of which were Ben Bradlee, editor of the *Washington Post,* and John F. Kennedy.[12] Later, women and persons of different ethnic and social groups were added, including the descendants of the original subjects.

The article states that Dr. George Vaillant, who led the study for thirty-five years and the author of at least three books on the subject, believes that aging successfully "is something like being tickled—it is achieved best with another person." Perhaps with the history of our generation affecting us, residences such as Planet X provide a welcome place in which to make this possible. We see each other almost every day, and our friendships can be deep and abiding. We grieve when we lose a beloved friend, but we have learned to accept it as the price of enjoying the friendship with one another. Writing this reminds me that we become close with those on the staff as well. I had to pick up our dinner last night because Husband had a cold; A., one of our wonderful servers, said, "Now you tell [Husband] to take care of himself and get well quick. We're thinking of him!" We all win when we open ourselves to one another. No, we cannot tickle ourselves.

There have been some unexpected, almost surprising results discovered from this intensive study. "I had expected that the longevity of your parents, the quality of your childhood, and your cholesterol levels would be very influential. So I was very surprised that these particular variables weren't more important than they were," said Dr. Vaillant.[13] His key takeaway is important: *"The seventy-five years and twenty million dollars expended on the Grant Study points … to a straightforward five-word conclusion: 'Happiness is love. Full stop.'"*[14]

Dr. Robert Waldinger, current director of the study, psychiatrist at Massachusetts General Hospital, and professor of psychiatry at Harvard

Medical School, later added: "The surprising finding is that our relationships and how happy we are in our relationships has a powerful influence on our health. *Taking care of your body is important, but tending to your relationships is a form of self-care too. That, I think, is the revelation.*"[15]

"When we gathered together everything we knew about them about at age 50, it wasn't their middle age cholesterol levels that predicted how they were going to grow old," said Waldinger in a popular TED Talk. "It was how satisfied they were in their relationships. The people who were the most satisfied in their relationships at age 50 were the healthiest at age 80."[16]

Surprisingly, the Harvard Study showed that stress was not a good predictor of poor health in old age. "Some people had a lot of stress, but aged very well. But *how you deal with that stress does matter quite a bit,*" says Dr. Vaillant.[17] Rather than obsessing about your cholesterol level or the genetic hand you were dealt, the study found that you'd be better off occupying yourself with these factors:

- avoiding cigarettes and alcohol;
- keeping a healthy weight;
- exercising regularly;
- pursuing education;
- maintaining strong social relationships, including a stable marriage; and
- developing good adjustment or coping skills—learning to make lemonade out of lemons.

After chatting with both of the women who recently had their 101st birthdays here at Planet X, I came away thinking they were both skilled at dealing with the lemons in their lives.

Even if your present lifestyle isn't what it should be, Dr. Vaillant believes it is never too late to change: "It's a little like opening an IRA. The earlier you start one, the better, but no matter what your age, it's still worth doing."[18]

Dr. V. believes that if we put aside brooding, and cultivate our curiosity and creativity, it will help transform older people into younger people. Individuals who maintain a playful spirit and find younger friends as they lose older ones are making the most of the aging process. Play is good for young children and for old children as well! Perhaps this justifies the bridge, poker, Scrabble, and other games that are so popular at Planet X.

The study also paid some attention to the fact that when we live alone we tend to eat less well, which may cause us to have a weaker immune system. *Depression and too much alcohol are also factors in early aging* due to their influence in keeping us from seeking out social contacts. But, although we do not want to overindulge in alcohol, let us not forget that a glass of wine a day is often recommended.

Now, I need to introduce you to Dr. William Thomas, author of *What Are Old People For? How Elders Will Save the World,* who asks us to consider the total structure of our society and to rethink old age. Dr. Thomas is responsible for one of the newer developments in elder care, the Eden Alternative,[19] an organization with a comforting and caring concept of older persons happily living with adults and animals, *engaged in meaningful activities ongoing from their life's past.* Dr. T. is perhaps one of the leading medical professionals seriously concerned with improving the quality of elderly life and how we are being served.

The Eden Alternative is not the only forward-thinking group associated with elder care, but it is currently the philosophy used in over three hundred homes in the United States. It is one example of a leading trend toward change in the care of elderly citizens, from "institutional models of care to person-directed values and practices that put the person first. Person-directed care is structured around the unique needs, preferences, and desires of each individual."[20] The values directing these programs include *choice, dignity, respect, self-determination, and purposeful living,* and the focus is on *eliminating the forces of loneliness, helplessness, and boredom,* which Dr. Thomas and the Eden Alternative identify as separate risk factors for adults.

There are many reasons for seniors to feel lonely, helpless, and bored. Loneliness is a subjective feeling of isolation, of not belonging, or lacking companionship that can occur despite proximity to others. Most of us have experienced feeling alone, even in a crowd, and it can be the cause of unhappiness, and even a decline in health for both older and younger people. However, the present institutional mindset of senior homes, often without meaning to, contributes to, rather than negates, the feeling of ineffectual aloneness, helplessness, and lack of importance in most decision-making processes. Last year when we were elected to the Residents Council, my friends and I were told by some older residents, "Don't expect to accomplish anything. It just won't happen." This is a dreadfully negative feeling with which to enter and live one's old age. It seems to deny that residents have any voice in how the large sums of money that we are paying to live in these homes are spent, and the assumption seems to be that we have turned our personhood over to the corporation. Not true! Not true! This attitude from corporate staff is a real turnoff to some seniors, causing them to stop trying to share their ideas and instead retreat to their apartment and a life of noninvolvement.

Despite our desire to be unique, feeling that we belong, as Dr. Vaillant tells us, is just as important as it was when we were young. *Belongingness is important for overall happiness, and depression comes when we feel that we don't belong.* I thought of this today when I received a draft copy of the cover of my new book (the one you're reading!). What did I do? I made a copy and ran down the hall to show it to my friend.

The other day I read a news article about a new church that was having its first service the following Sunday. What intrigued me was the name of the church. One simple, descriptive word: *Belong*. I must admit I was hooked. I would have been in the front pew had this group of worshipers been close enough for me to attend. I'd love it if we could change the name of our senior home to Belong: *to belong one has to believe that one contributes to his or her home and is not just a user of available facilities.*

Another avenue to happiness at any age is being helpful to others, which recent research has shown brings us more joy than does helping ourselves. It's no surprise that many movements of what we might call the enlightenment emphasized the *importance of showing concern for others and involving oneself in activities that transcend the self.* (Two role models come to mind: Martin Luther King Jr. and the Dalai Lama.) It isn't that other people need "fixing." We all have strengths and something unique to offer. It is simply that we are at our best when we receive validation and feel a part of what is happening in our world. Judgments build walls. Giving tumbles them.

In one of his last books, *Recessional*, author James Michener points to a recent widow in his fictional retirement community who is grieving and feeling lost. In this story, the community director goes to the widow's apartment and spends time simply sitting with and comforting her. In my experience, staff seldom or never seem to have time for this. They may voice a passing remark or pat a shoulder, but then they must be off to do today's business as outlined by Corporate. However, time spent one-on-one with residents, comforting them and making them feel like they belong here, incorporating Eden Alternative principles, would pay dividends in the long run and perhaps do a lot to help the widow find a reworked future. I have to admit, however, that it need not just be staff who would do this—it could be just as helpful coming from a fellow resident.

I encourage everyone to learn more about the Eden Alternative, which you can do by visiting its website.[21] It is just one indication of a breakthrough toward better and more understanding care for elders. Perhaps in the future, instead of being infantilized and not included in decision-making, elders will be able to have a greater voice in the simple things of their daily life and to live in a community where *friendship and relationships are everyday things.*

Dr. Thomas also opened my eyes to something I had only halfway realized: America's excessive dedication to adult power has caused both children and elders to have serious identity problems within the adult society. Rather than be considered of value in themselves, children are expected to grow into adulthood as quickly as possible. The wunderkind mimics adult behaviors, and the best child is the most precocious child, just as those elders whom adults consider the most worthy are the ones who defy their older age and continue to work, talk, look like, and think like adults—in other words, those elders who desperately fight the natural act of aging. "In the studies I have made," Dr. Thomas says, *"there is an alternate role for seniors in which they don't have to act in the same way younger persons do."*[22]

I think of Joan Rivers and the extensive plastic surgery done, I believe, to fit into a world that panics at the thought of getting old. I so wish she could have been as humorous to the adult American by just aging naturally, but I doubt that could have happened. It is distressing to see older persons spend life's resources trying to remain young. It is useless to aggressively quest for the physical beauty and influences of our younger years. It is not useless, nor is it unattainable, to use one's resources to make elderhood a vital, fruitful, rich time of our lives, one that has its own responsibilities and duties. And joys. More on that later.

My mother dyed her hair until she entered the Alzheimer's unit at age eighty-three. I have a few friends here who cannot bear the thought of letting their hair return to its natural white, but most of us have whitened out quite nicely, thank you. I think boomers are even less afraid of white hair. My daughter went white at thirty, and many of her friends are doing the same. They proudly sport their gray hair in quite sophisticated styles, looking beautiful as they age naturally.

To summarize: adulthood fashions its outlook with a desire to make both children and seniors into its own image. This shortens the so-called useful life to about forty-four years, since usefulness would not start until one is about twenty-one and legal, and then one would not have any convincing usefulness or importance after sixty-five. This makes no sense. Let us insist that a functional life be extended well beyond any arbitrary age.

Contrarily, Dr. Thomas believes that although adulthood is a vital, interesting, and important part of a person's, and a society's, life, it is unhealthy for a society to expect its children to be miniature adults, or its elders to scramble to maintain a false façade and to believe that their senior age has nothing to offer. Instead, he urges us to visualize a richer elder life for ourselves by *finding a sense of purpose*, stating, "Purpose reflects a commitment to broader life goals that helps organize your day to day activities."[23] Some other words that I use for this human drive are *motivation, focus,* and *incentive.*

Regardless of age, having a sense of purpose is a necessity for a full life and is associated with satisfaction, happiness, better physical functioning, and even better sleep, or so say the experts. I have asked fellow residents what purpose they have and, unfortunately, very often I get a blank look in response. This is not a criticism of my friends; it is just that, even though they might have a very useful purpose in their lives, it has never been something that many of us have focused on. Possibly they haven't thought of their purpose in those words, but having one is "a very robust predictor of health and wellness in old age,"[24] says Dr. Patricia Boyle, a neuropsychologist at the Rush Alzheimer's Disease Center in Chicago, quoted in the *New York Times* article "Living on Purpose."

I know that when I am enthused about my writing and other projects, I forget my aches and pains. I get out of my apartment more, move around more, and can feel my mind racing to keep up with me. I feel happy and of value at these times. How could that not be beneficial to my health? Yes, I can so enthusiastically identify with Dr. Boyle's words. Although I have a bad back, when I'm feeling purposeful I can walk for a reasonable distance. And just today, I bounced into the dining room feeling ten years younger. Why? I had been working on this book and all was going well. That joy feels so good, and I know it looks good, too!

In their study of purpose, Dr. Boyle's research team tracked two groups of elders (approximately one thousand participants) living independently in Chicago, assessing them regularly using a variety of measures. What did they find? First, *those with high purpose scores were 2.4 times more likely to remain free of Alzheimer's than those with low scores, and they were less likely to have mild cognitive impairment.* Per Dr. Boyle, *having a sense of purpose* (a high purpose score in this study) "also *slowed the rate of cognitive decline by about 30 percent.*"[25] Thirty percent! That is significant. (To have a sense of purpose is itself a purpose, and being mentally active increases our chances of maintaining cognitive excellence. Because I watched my mother and my husband deal with dementia, one purpose I have in engaging in my activities is to try to avoid it for myself.)

Autopsies of 246 persons from Dr. Boyle's group showed that *many of those who felt they were leading a purposeful life, and who displayed no sign of Alzheimer's or impairment, had the plaques and tangles expected in Alzheimer's patients.* Why, then, had they not developed Alzheimer's? Dr. Boyle concluded that *purposeful living allowed them to tolerate the plaque and brain tangles of Alzheimer's and still maintain an intelligent mode of life.*

Wow!

Dr. Boyle's research team also found that purposeful people were less likely to develop disabilities or to die. In a sample group followed for up to five years (average age seventy-eight), *those with high purpose had roughly half the mortality rate of those with low purpose.*

The article "Living on Purpose" also discusses the work of Dr. Patrick Hill of Carleton University in Ottawa, who looked at whether purpose has less power over human health after retirement, when, according to Dr. Hill, "you're starting to lose those structures you had, a natural way to organize your daily life."[26] Somewhat to Dr. Hill's surprise, work status didn't matter. This says to me that purposeful people are purposeful people who continue to find a function for life aside from their life's work and regardless of their age.

Another article I read, this one on ScienceDaily.com, supports Dr. Boyle's findings on purpose and mortality. Drs. Randy Cohen and Alan Rozanski and colleagues at Mount Sinai St. Luke's-Roosevelt Hospital in New York pooled data from ten previous studies that evaluated the relationship between purpose in life and the risk of death or cardiovascular disease. Data on more than 136,000 participants, mainly from the United States or Japan, were analyzed. The analysis showed that participants with a strong sense of purpose in life had a lower risk of death, about one-fifth lower. The researchers also found that *a strong sense of purpose is related to a lower risk of cardiovascular events.*[27]

I have seen purpose at work here at Planet X. A wonderful, interesting gentleman in his nineties who exercised thirty minutes every day and had a loving family seemed to suddenly lose his zeal, his purpose in his life. Within six months he died. I yearn to know why he stopped caring. He had been prone to bragging to everyone that he exercised religiously. His routine was broken up by a change in the exercise equipment availability, and I have wondered if losing that may have thrown him into depression. It is possible that losing that daily challenge caused him to feel unmotivated and unhealthy. In his later days, I would see him sitting and doing nothing for long stretches of time. This was very unlike the man I knew when we first moved into Planet X.

However, we never know the depths of another's mind, do we? Every now and then I see people, like F., who seem to choose to live no longer. I'm not sure what happens when one reaches that time, but sometimes the body seems to know when it is the end, and when it is the end, even purpose is not what one is thinking about. We will all have an end time, and purpose will take us just so far.

An example of ongoing purpose is a letter I read from the Ask Amy column in the *Chicago Tribune.* I had placed the clipping in my files because, I think, it spoke to me, even at an earlier age. The woman who wrote the letter said that, like another person who wrote in, she, too, has trouble with regrets for past actions, but then one day she remembered something Ghandi had said: "Be the change I want to see in the world." At that point it occurred to her that she could apply this concept when she feels a regret and that, although it doesn't change the past, she feels better knowing she is moving forward "being the change."[28]

Attitude toward life is another human trait that has been researched in relation to aging. It turns out that *how we view the world around us has a significant influence on how our old age progresses.* As reported in a *Wall Street Journal* Health Matters article, Dr. Becca Levy and colleagues at Yale University reviewed surveys taken by 386 men and women in 1968 when they were under age fifty, and then again nearly four decades later, as part of the Baltimore Longitudinal Study of Aging. Of those who in 1968 believed older people were feeble, helpless, absent-minded, and make too many mistakes, 25 percent had cardiovascular events in their later years, as contrasted with the more positive group, of which only 13 percent had such events.[29] This is a significant difference.

I took a minute just now to ask myself how I see myself and my life. My answer is that I'm not too happy with the physical beauty of me, but I know that I still have a lot of life to live inside of my decrepit outer face. But that's me. If you are over sixty-five, how do you see yourself? As a society, in politics, and as members of an aging group, we dwell so much on personal appearance that it becomes easy to miss our other talents and excellence, and even the joys in our life. This is what is meant when we tell someone we're beautiful inside. Such an attitude can affect our later years, according to Dr. Levy and colleagues.

In an earlier study Dr. Levy found that *660 persons over age fifty who in 1975 viewed aging as a positive experience lived an average of 7.5 years longer than those with negative views.*[30] Talk about a self-fulfilling prophesy. If you have a positive attitude about your age and believe that old people can be active, vital, and healthy members of society, you may take better care of yourself than if you believe you are on a slow slide into the grave.

In other articles we are given an indication of Dr. Levy's concerns: "I've become more sensitive to observing the kind of language people use to talk about aging in general, their own aging, and that of other people they encounter."[31] Levy says that patronizing attitudes and speaking to elders as if they were children ("elderspeak") can affect both competence and lifespan: *"Those little insults can lead to more negative images of aging. And those who have more negative images of aging have worse functional health over time, including lower rates of survival."*[32] She also suggests that stereotypes of aging in our culture may go farther than just making us feel bad: *"Negative images of aging could be a public health issue,"* she says.[33]

Other studies by Dr. Levy, discussed in her journal article "Mind Matters: Cognitive and Physical Effects of Aging Self-Stereotypes," found that older participants exposed subliminally to negative stereotype words such as *decrepit* did worse on memory tests, had shakier handwriting, and were less steady on their feet than those who were exposed to positive stereotype words such as *wisdom.*[34] This says something about the attitudes of those who care for us in our later years. If we see negatives about ourselves, or our age, reflected from others or in their eyes, it can cause us to react negatively to our own lives. Levy believes that *positive attitudes that translate into better memory, and a longer life, might have something to do with the will to live and a belief that the positives in life outweigh the negatives.* And she has a sensitivity to how seniors see themselves:

"I hate the term 'senior moment'—I just hate it," she says. "Because if you start to use terms like that about yourself, even if you're kidding, it's going to have a negative impact on your self-esteem."[35] Few of us can argue with Dr. Levy's findings.

I must compliment most of the staff here at Planet X. I am never made to feel decrepit, even though I sometimes think that things are done more to me and for me rather than with me. And I am seldom aware that they see us as geezers or look at us in an uninterested way. We are treated with friendship and respect, and we are not talked to as though we were babies. Occasionally a staff member who has had no experience working with seniors simply doesn't like it here and quits. I often wonder if it is because that person feels uncomfortable talking with older persons.

Fortunately, we have help in our efforts to live deeply: magically the human body has a potential energy source within which can make us stronger or weaker as we age. As reported in the article "Protein Protects Aging Brain" about a study conducted by Harvard Medical School, this energy source was found in a class of protein substances that can protect our neurons against injury and death. These substances can stimulate the production of new neurons from adult stem cells in the brain. What is to be remembered about this bit of information is that the stimulation and production of this protein is influenced by the amount of activity going on in nearby neural circuits.[36] As Dr. Nuland says, "Those who continue to challenge themselves are likely to be those who maintain the capacity to do so."[37]

For me, the message is: do something, anything. Don't just sit there. As my daughter says, sitting is the new smoking, and is just as hazardous to our physical and mental health. Our good health requires movement, learning, and activity to keep the mind making new neurons. *Dullness, negativity, and lethargy are lethal to the older mind.*

Concern for what components lead to successful aging is not limited to American studies. For example, in Seoul, South Korea, research on what makes up successful aging was completed in 2016. The researchers found that successful aging rests on four components:

1. avoiding disease and disability;
2. having high cognitive/mental/physical functioning;

3. actively engaging in life; and
4. working to be psychologically well adapted to later life.[38]

The study was done to provide evidence for building interventions for the aging South Korean population. Let us hope that American planners are as wise.

An analysis of life expectancy in all parts of the world was done by the National Institutes of Health (the NIH) and published in the book *The Blue Zones: Lessons for Living Longer from the People Who've Lived the Longest* by Dan Buettner. Blue Zone longevity pockets include Sardinia, Italy, and Okinawa, Japan, and other areas where the life expectancy is the best in the world. In the book, Buettner lists the "Power 9"—nine characteristics of the Blue Zone lifestyle of elders:

1. *Move naturally.* Create a lifestyle that includes active living.
2. *Purpose.* Have a reason to get up in the morning.
3. *Downshift.* Build stress reduction into your routines, such as napping, happy hour, and daily prayer.
4. *80% rule.* Stop eating when you are 80% full; eat your largest meal midday and the smallest meal later in the day.
5. *Plant slant.* Beans, such as fava, black, soy, and lentils, are the cornerstone of most centenarian diets; meat, mostly pork, is eaten on average only five times per month.
6. *Wine @ 5.* People in most of the zones drink alcohol moderately and regularly.
7. *Belong.* Belonging to a faith-based community is common in the zones.
8. *Loved ones first.* Putting family first is a common element.
9. *Right tribe.* Lifestyle habits are often caught, not taught; long-lived people's health behaviors have been favorably shaped by their social networks.[39]

Worth noting is the absence of any mention of medication. *It is all about lifestyle.* Perhaps we can build our own Blue Zone here at Planet X. So many of us are flooded with medicines, and we are grateful to have them if they keep us healthy. However, I keep asking my doctor what I must do to get rid of some of them. Sometimes it is only a matter of losing weight and getting exercise. We may not get off the med entirely, but we may be able to lower the dosage.

We old folks aren't so different from what we were like when we were young, and some of us are really good at avoiding living a healthy lifestyle. It's too much trouble, we tell ourselves. Exercise is always something that a responsible physician will recommend. However, in *The Art of Aging,* Dr. Sherwin Nuland shares the dissenting opinion of Dr. Leo Cooney, who founded the Section of Geriatrics at the Yale School of Medicine: "Exercise is not the Holy Grail. If there's a Holy Grail, it's relationships with other people. In fact, if you have to decide between going to the gym or being with your grandchildren, I'd choose the grandchildren."[40] Age does not, or should not, separate us from our social encirclements, but, rather, to stimulate the desire to live fully, we need to enhance these relationships with exercise and nutrition.

Viktor Frankl reiterates again and again in his book *Man's Search for Meaning* that if we humans lose all else, we still have that last freedom—the freedom to "choose one's attitude in a given set of circumstances."[41] This knowledge dates back to the ancient Stoic philosophers and is the foundation of humankind's resilience today. We cannot choose whether to be old, but we can choose our attitude and the resolve with which we wish to live these remaining years. We can even decide whether to listen to the researchers or ignore them and continue to live as we wish.

How we spend our days is, of course, how we spend our lives.

—ANNIE DILLARD, *THE WRITING LIFE*

SEVEN

Reflecting on the Mountain

> It is after we get home that we really go over the mountain, if ever. What did the mountain say? What did the mountain do?
> —HENRY DAVID THOREAU, IN AN 1857 LETTER TO HARRISON G. O. BLAKE

Reflecting on our thirty-eight months at Planet X, our mountain, has required me to reexamine a myriad of assumptions I have held about life, about aging, and about places like Planet X. I admit that my months of study have caused me to think about what Paulo Coelho spoke of in *The Alchemist:* living life with "the language of enthusiasm, of things accomplished with love and purpose, and as part of a search for something believed in and desired."[1] As I returned to look once again at my newish home, I wondered if in this last third of our lives there really is any good way for our society to provide a solid backdrop where those older members who desire to do so might, perhaps for the first time, discover Coelho's enthusiasm, love, and purpose in their lives.

My first assumptions about living in a senior center were typically skewed. Even though I had old person experience from my parents' last years, my life's book did not include the kind of useful information I needed to evaluate how today one can successfully and fully live that last third of life, especially in a senior residence. It certainly did not tell me what tomorrow might bring for the baby boomers.

Here at Planet X I have met those, some of whom have found their personal legend, as Coelho calls it, who are peacefully getting old and following the precepts they have been taught by their church or by example, while others have self-discovered the secret to finding purpose and enthusiasm for living their life thoroughly till the end. As in any communal setting some here are discontent, but given the encouragement of friends and staff, perhaps there is a chance that they, too, can find peace and meaning in these last years. I am convinced that these years have a purpose, but it is always a personal challenge for each of us to embark on a singular journey to find meaning in our own life. If our mountain, Planet X, could talk, it might say, "Here is a place where you can work out your dreams, care for your illnesses, have understanding and help if needed, and live or even discover the final meaning of your life if you have the desire to do so."

That is the dream, but how does one weave it into his or her life at Planet X? I can credit my friend Henry Thoreau for describing how we can look more intelligently at the mountains we experience in life. He encourages us to, after the climb, look carefully at the complete experience, mull it over, and then try to apply what we have learned to the remainder of our life. I know that I'm sincerely pleased that I took the time to do some research about this mountain of old age instead of accepting my first negative reactions to the pain of the move, our new home, and the experience of aging itself.

You, Dear Reader, will have to judge how much weight to put on the research and opinions noted and espoused here, for I am only one American soul. There is a lot of aging research available, and there will undoubtedly be a lot more. It is said one can prove anything by research, but let me assure you that, if nothing else, my search has given me, personally, a healthier outlook with which to live my remaining years.

Now that I am back from my research jaunt in chapter 6, we'll take a look at Planet X, I'll introduce you to my friends, and hopefully you will come away with a better picture of senior residences than I painted shortly after I arrived here. Planet X is an excellent example of contemporary care residences in America, and how we are living here at this present moment may suggest even more creative ideas for senior life in the future. We are not speaking here of extended care for those who are bedridden or in a memory care unit. Here at Planet X we can get help, hire help, and be helped, but we are continually reminded that this is "independent" living.

As we begin to look carefully at the communal home in which my friends and I live, I warn the critics that successful aging takes thought and planning and money, and its faults cannot be completely laid at the feet of the senior care corporations or those they hire. It starts with the individual, and much of the success or failure of aging, now and in the future, is on the doorstep of we agers ourselves, and, by default, our families. How we feel about living here is closely tied to what we accept as the truth about our personal lives.

There is a tendency on the part of some elderly residents—perhaps because our society has groomed them for the role—to feel that they are paying to be cared for, and the slide to inactivity or noninvolvement in the activities of our home can be swift and sure for those who view aging as a time to rest, and not be bothered. When such attitudes are seen by Corporate, there is little wonder that the institution takes over. Someone must run things. Traditionally that is who we hired to do the job. If we elders want to be seen as off the shelf, we have to want to climb off the shelf and get the physical or emotional help necessary to know what we need and want. We cannot be forgiven if we create the shelf ourselves by sitting back, not being available, and not seeing ourselves as capable, reliable, creative folks who are interested in determining at least some of the details of our final years.

If we are afraid of our own aging, or have difficulty working around the obvious ills and misfortunes of our years, others will tell us who we are and what we should be doing. This may be what we think we want, but I doubt that that is true for the majority of older Americans. Perhaps some of us are victims of society's advertising, but let us think bigger than that.

Getting old isn't easy, but it can be extremely rewarding, given a purposeful mindset and a willing attitude. The most difficult thought to accept is that there is no answer for these years that is right for everyone, regardless of what any expert says. Aging will be different for each individual, but there are, at least collectively, a few things that will make life richer and even in some cases longer: (1) socialization, (2) finding a sense of purpose, and (3) trying hard to keep a positive attitude. These are good places to start according to some of the research we've seen.

Let's start with socialization. Living alone in one's home automatically makes it more difficult to be around others. One must motivate the old self and either entertain others or get the old bones going and go out to meet said friends.

At Planet X social opportunities abound and are right at hand. Let me share a very touching story of two people, friends of mine in their eighties or nineties. I'm not trying to publicize for romance in elder centers, but consider this story taking into account the benefits of socialization.

I never really asked their age; it was their life here at Planet X that brought tears to my eyes. It was their friendship and love that offers an example of why I say that we are responsible for the direction of our own aging. And I am eager for you to meet them. Their experience is a beautiful example of why life need not be over at sixty-five.

Place yourself in a chair in the lobby of Planet X. There are bouquets of flowers, and a picture of an elderly gentleman with the dates of his birth and death. (When there is a death at Planet X, it is common for the family to share their grief with us, the friends, in the form of a short memorial service.) After the opening music and a heartfelt eulogy by the gentleman's son, my friend C. stood up and quietly began to speak. C. is allowing me to share here the story she told.

I would like to share with you a short story, actually, a short love story. It began right here in this room one Friday afternoon at a wine social. I came in and sat down next to a very sweet gentleman. I didn't find out just how sweet until later. He introduced himself as B. and offered to get me a glass of wine. I told him my name was C., thanked him, and said I would get my own wine. B. was using a walker, and I thought it was easier if I got my own wine.

B. loved the Friday afternoon wine socials. He liked to swing back and forth with the music and would twirl me around even as he sat. On Valentine's Day I saw him in the lobby. As I walked by I said, "Happy Valentine's Day, B." He stood up and said, "I want to give you a hug." I said, "OK," and he gave me a great big hug.

The next time I saw him, he asked me out for Sunday brunch. I thought, how sweet. It had been over sixty years since someone had asked me for a date. I hoped I would remember how to behave. Going out for brunch became a regular thing, and we enjoyed being together. B. liked sports, so I used to go to his apartment and watch baseball, boxing, and football with him. We would have a bottle of beer or a glass of wine. Oh, how B. loved his wine. He also liked to watch game shows. I would surprise him (and myself) when I came up with the answers to some of the questions. He would ask, "How did you know that?" and I would answer, "I know stuff."

Soon it was obvious this was more than friendship. We had become sweethearts. We talked about marriage, but B. said he was too old to get married, and I said I didn't want to get married either. I just wanted someone to treat me nice and do nice things for me. He said, "I can do that," and the next thing I knew I was wearing a sweetheart ring. He was always doing nice things for me. One time when the boutique came to sell things in the lobby, he called and said, "You better get down here and pick out something you like." How sweet is that?

C. paused, looked down, took a deep breath, then said softly, "Even though the story has come to an end, the love never will."

There was not a sound in the room as C. finished. I sat there with tears in my eyes as my friend spoke. We understood: we understood the friendship, the depth of feeling and understanding they had shared, and we understood the undefinable meaning that such a relationship can give to an aging couple. With composure, acceptance, and love, C. then sang their favorite love song, and as she sang, we cried. We cried the tears of the aged, which are different from the tears of youth.

Friends, this is old age at its most poignant—brought about by two people not confining themselves in their apartments or homes, but being available for companionship and experiences offered as a part of our community life here at Planet X. Love, friendship, and companionship in so many of their semblances are here for the asking. They disclose themselves in so many different ways as we aging mortals come together. We just have to look for them and accept them as they present themselves. Humans are, at heart, groupies, and we thrive when we can accept that and feel comfortable in the group, even if that group is only one other person. It is easy to chuckle when one sees a couple walking through our halls holding hands, or sitting arm in arm in the fading light, but consider: Why does caring and concern have to end when one has gray hair? Why are tender feelings, regardless of age, something to scorn or find embarrassing?

C. often mentions her lost love to us, but she has not gone into mourning or lost interest in her life. She participates in our singing group here and in her church choir, is a member of her church circle, plays bridge, and is president of our Residents Council.

As I introduce you to our aging universe, however, I don't wish to tell you of only the victories, the high points, for there is also sadness, loss, the pain of change and of losing friends, and the sting of knowing that some of these losses could possibly have been avoided until a later time if changes in lifestyle or environment had been made (or so the research is telling us). Lives snuffed early due to negative attitudes, loneliness, lack of medical care, and stubborn depression are with us as well.

Yes, we see our friends and loved ones pass before our eyes, and even our own health is something that must be handled cautiously. At times, just taking care of that seems to consume our days. Know, however, that it is worth it. Granted that this last third of life can be extremely rewarding and revealing, but it requires the ability to look beyond the negatives.

Planet X provides us with friendship, companionship, and time for fun and conversation, but there is also the piano. Let me explain. A large grand piano graces the lobby of Planet X, and we always enjoy its melodies when played at special times. However, it symbolizes another side of life: whenever a friend dies, a picture of that person with his or her name and dates of birth and death is placed on the piano—usually accompanied by a bouquet of blossoms. Life is both lived and lost at Planet X, and the piano tells the tale. This final stage of life requires an acceptance of "the piano and its song."

But I am ahead of myself. I have been asked why anyone should move from a beloved private home to a senior residence. What does one get from the distress of such a painful move? Well, like my friend A., I'm glad we're here. Let me share A.'s story.

A. is one of those who gives Planet X some of its sunshine. A.'s friend G. has recently had a bad turn of health, so A. had to move him from Planet X to a special group home where he could get more care than she could provide here. (Having to make such a move is not unusual for many of us here. As the body we live with weakens, we must find rehabilitation, assisted living, or another living situation.) The two have been extremely close for several years, and now, with G.'s family in nonattendance, A. is his power of attorney caregiver and loved one. The grief of moving him falls back on A., and A. alone.

A.'s words here clearly indicate what this place means to her. We were sharing experiences in our women's group and were touched when she shook her head, teared up a little, and said, "Thank you, friends. You just don't know how glad I am that I'm able to come home and feel the comfort. I am so very happy I live here with all of you."

Putting aside any differences we might have with Planet X Corporation, almost all of us agree that it is better to be with our friends and the staff we know and care for than to be alone. This just must be what the social scientists mean when they speak of the need for socialization. No, we cannot tickle ourselves, and finally, at this advanced age, we are able to admit how much our friendships mean to us. We are losing our one-anothers all the time, making those who remain that much more precious. Research says it and our lives prove it: we need our friends in this latter stage of life. As C. said, the love remains. We remember and we care.

We have talked of socialization, but let us take a closer look at the social networking that occurs in a place like Planet X. Small talk is rampant here, but I have come to realize that it serves a purpose by helping us get to know others without risking deeper beliefs and branding ourselves as on one side or another as we struggle to find our niche. (Our generation doesn't open up to just anyone, you know.) Some of us even get to the stage of friendship where we can discuss politics or religion. One friend and I are very aware that we cancel out each other's vote at every election, but we've gotten beyond the anger that that can bring to lesser friends. We fuss, we argue, then we part and say, "See you tomorrow." Another friend and I have vowed that we will not let a petty spat spoil our friendship. I don't think I have ever had better friends. I've had more friends, but not better ones.

When we first moved to Planet X, I was critical of what seemed to be superficial dialogue, wondering if small talk was all we have to offer to one another. "How are you?" "How's it going?" Et cetera. I wondered if I would ever get to really know anyone well enough to have an in-depth conversation, but I had forgotten that small talk is a necessary prologue to friendship, especially considering that most of us were unacquainted prior to moving to Planet X. I have since found a new respect for chitchat. It proves to be an important first step in moving a relationship on to bigger attachments. It's a bit like dipping one's toe in the water.

Silly, but this reminds me of last night when Lucy, our dog, and I took an early evening stroll. We met a new resident, M., who couldn't find her way around the building to her apartment. M.'s dog and Lucy looked at one another, sniffed a bit, touched noses, and then Lucy did her terrier prance on all fours, as though to say, "You're OK. Let's play!" Her new friend's tail began to wag—she understood Lucy's friendly gesture I guess—and they began their doggie play in earnest. I couldn't help but draw a comparison between this and how we humans here sniff out one another. For some it's an easy sniff, but what if some of us are barkers, or even biters? This reminds me of an issue I wanted to mention. Let's take this metaphor a bit further. If this is a place where the emphasis is on the person, not the institution, then we must remember that there is Doodles, our resident Pekingese, who chooses to hide between her owner's legs when another dog approaches. Yes, some of us here are shy, or introverted. But these people pay their monthly rent like everyone else and still count and need to be attended to.

So, does Planet X have a responsibility when it takes our rent to exhibit a greater concern for the individual, and should part of its service be to benefit the Doodleses of this senior residence as well as those of us who have no trouble capering and playing with one another? We all pay Corporate like sums of money, and something that may need to be considered in the future is that these differences in personality are the way of the world, forever and anon. Activities and plans for the care for all should be a part of Corporate's plan of encouragement—and should include helping the Doodles as well as the Lucys who have chosen senior living. If socialization and feeling part of a group are advantageous to our health, I ask, does this then become a task of the senior care giver, to make a sincere effort to help the individual reach that goal? Is offering classes and activities enough? Some who stay in their apartment most of the time may like it that way. Others are, I know, too ill to come out to socialize, or too shy. Or are they lonely and possibly bored? I don't know if anyone bothers to find out.

This makes me aware that there is no counseling available to residents. I know that many of us are needing to talk things over with someone. We have a Planet X group that provides help with bathing, walking the dog, shopping, etc. But no counseling. Boomers are going to be looking for such nuances, I would judge. If, as research indicates, socialization is life-giving, it should, in various modes, be indicated for all. I myself would like to see more attention given to such subtleties. With such a large population at our residence, some of our more inward elders get lost. There are some who are thrown off by the fuss made about where one sits in the dining room; for others it's "Who will talk to me since I've had that stroke and can't speak well?" or "My hearing is bad so no one pays attention to me." Some of these friends peek from their doorways only on occasion.

I know our program director has said that her main concern is getting people out of their rooms. It is, of course, an attitude that all senior and junior staff members should put as a priority, not just the program director, if, indeed, socialization is as important to the health of aging individuals as research shows. Instead of spending so much of the time doing nonpersonal work, it seems more beneficial to seniors for staff to put people first and computer work second. Too often a senior staffer is found mainly in his or her office.

They are closeted there and are available if called forth by the concierge, or if we happen to catch them in the halls. Availability to residents seems to me to be too limited. Residents would like to see them eating in our dining room and involving themselves in some of the activities. The executive director that we had a year ago was not above cleaning a room if help was short and often poured coffee in the dining room, chatting with residents.

What seems to draw senior women out and into the fold are small groups that meet to discuss topics meaningful to them personally: family, values, and even hopes and dreams. And then there are the men: their morning gabfests over breakfast are sacred, and I am told they go into great depth about football, baseball, and even politics. One cannot measure the value of such discussions, but they do let us "tickle one another," as Dr. Vaillant might say. I hope in the future to see more effort to get residents working together creatively. Joint projects always seems to help us form friendships. Our writing group, the gardening group, the jewelry group are all creative groups that encourage friendships. We have just started a newsletter that is drawing more and more residents and staff to contribute articles, ideas, and pictures. There is something very positive in a resident coming up to me and saying, "Here, put this in our newsletter." Yes, it is *our* newsletter.

Of course most of us had neighborhood friends before moving here, but here at Planet X, due to how close we live to one another, it should be even easier to befriend others: we may see someone two, three, four times a day. We have similar problems and mindsets, and without our really realizing it, this brings us together. And we become very aware of those who are missing. I heard last night that L. had been rushed to the hospital with a possible stroke. The network went to work, with no help from the concierge, to check with family and friends and scope out the truth of her illness. A few minutes later the phone lines buzzed and chatter went forth that R. had also been taken to the hospital, with some undetermined problem. The messages flew from table to table at dinner, informing one and all about these current worries and giving us some idea about what is going on. I've often wished that one of us would take it as a purpose project to keep track of where our friends are and how their health is progressing.

Such contact and concern are hard to find in today's legally determined world. We need the residents' underground network. There are privacy laws that make knowing about a friend's health or current condition difficult.

But never fear; our news line is not always accurate, but it is faster than one might imagine: "Did you see C. sitting with B. at lunch?" "Yes, and did you hear that D. fell and broke her hip this morning when she reached for the phone?" The community newswire is always working. One can almost hear the lines clicking.

So how does Planet X help us with our attempts at friend making? What opportunities do we have at our disposal to grow close? Friday happy hour, for one. I told you about my initial hesitancy about happy hour. But I've been here a while now, so let me describe how good it is for some residents.

Happy hour is well attended here and a delight for many residents. Sometimes our relatives come, and everyone enjoys the food and drink. Residents dress up a little and head for the lobby at about four o'clock, and the music begins. I love to see the gray heads bob around as residents dance to the tunes of the oldies played on a wheezy accordion. They are living, and so are those who simply watch and smile. N. unhooks her oxygen line, jumps on the floor, and hops like a bouncing doll to "Hey! Ba-Ba-Re-Bop." She may have to grab a chair and fan herself afterward, but that never seems to stop her. N. loves life and all it offers and is willing to suffer a little to accommodate her passions. We who watch cross our fingers and hope the exercise is good for her. Some of us prefer to head for the hors d'oeuvres, while others gather in circles and begin the evening conversation. Unfortunately, a few residents are choosy about whom they connect with and will put reserved signs on tables in a show of exclusivity. This is not authorized by Planet X and fortunately most residents avoid this approach, but in a communal world all things are possible.

And then there is mealtime. It is amazing how much importance lunch and dinner play in our day. These are times for us to catch up with friends, sharing our lives and interests. "What did you do this a.m.?" "What's happening?" "How's your back this morning?" Not the conversation of youth, but it's all ours. My dear husband, even with his dementia, still loves to get it on with his cronies and whisper jokes we women aren't supposed to hear. He is well liked, and friends come by our table to kid him, giving him a hand slap and a high five now and then.

There was one old fellow I loved, gone now, who would wheel up in his peepmobile,[2] take a card from his pocket, and tell a silly joke. He couldn't remember the jokes, but he had them written down and just had to remain the life of the party. We obediently laughed even though it may have been the tenth time we heard said joke, but consider what this simple act did: it added humor to his and our lives, it gave him a social link to others, and it was a good way for him to keep a positive attitude and a sense of purpose. He was doing his part to keep our world happy.

Then there are the times when one of us makes a favorite dessert and invites a few friends in to enjoy, or when our good friend S. invites us for spaghetti and meatballs and proves he is a fabulous cook. Some of us trade DVDs and recipes we will probably never use, share news clippings and thoughts, gossip a little bit (more than a little bit), and have occasions to have genuinely happy times together. The pleasure of these years is built on the foundation, the very real idea, that each of us recognizes the beauty of each day and the joy of being able to revel in it. This love of *now* is a feeling we all share with one another, and our chatting, our jokes, our interest in health, and our working together on projects are all a part of how important our today really is.

So much of what I have been relating only reinforces what researchers are fostering: they are telling me that one way I can keep these priceless years from turning into a maudlin, self-pitying swamp is to watch my attitude and concentrate on how to keep the day-to-day joy of life. This isn't much of a surprise. Almost any age is made better by doing so, or made worse if all I choose to do is see the negative side of life, unable to convince myself to maintain a mindset that makes life richer for myself and others. Not only do I need others, but I need to look forward and not let self-pity or anger restrain my evolvement. Communal homes such as Planet X present us all with opportunities to grow and learn. (And they could be even more encouraging than they currently are, but more on that later.)

Which tells me that this is a good place to introduce our dear friend D. I will always see her approaching us with a smile from ear to ear, giving my husband a customary high five and telling us about how her tomato garden is growing. Few here do much gardening, but D., with only a little help from Corporate, has a good-sized patch out by her apartment, which she waters, tends, hoes, and loves. Her enthusiasm for her little patch has encouraged others who have joined her to make the garden a real community effort. I don't know of anyone who shares more of the joy of life with others than D., whom

I love dearly. She has added so much to my life. With friends like D., our world becomes richer by simply being in their shadow.

> Depth is found in what we can learn from the people and things around us. Everyone, everything has a story.... When you learn those stories, you learn experiences that fill you up, that expand your understanding. You add layers to your soul.
>
> —KASIE WEST, *THE FILL-IN BOYFRIEND*

I am learning that part of this time of my life is to see opportunities for friendship and growth where I might not expect to find them. I am reminded of a Hindu story Dr. Rachel Naomi Remen passed on in her book *Kitchen Table Wisdom: Stories That Heal,* about the god Shiva, who at the request of his wife, Shakti, drops a bag of gold in the path of a miserably poor man as he walks along, although he knows that the man is not ready to receive it. Seeing the bag of gold but thinking it is a rock that might have torn his sandals, the poor man carefully steps over it and goes on his away.

Dr. Remen, who counsels cancer patients, writes:

> It seems that Life drops many bags of gold in our path. Rarely do they look like what they are. I asked my patient if Life has ever dropped him a bag of gold that he has recognized and used to enrich his life. He smiles at me. "Cancer," he says simply. "I thought you'd guess."

Indeed, our old age is a bag of gold if we care to see it as so, and here at Planet X we are provided with an environment that encourages us to find that bag of gold. I personally am living my old age time, finding it to be a beautiful time of serious reflection on what has been and what should have been, and finding that life at this age can be a great deal of fun and a time of accomplishment. Coupling that with the idea that we have a second chance to leave good feelings to those who follow us makes it a win-win time we can use to our best advantage. How are we so lucky? Yes, this old age can, indeed, be our bag of gold.

Nevertheless, I acknowledge that not all elders see it as I do, and I admit that there are times when I find it difficult to look at my age as a bag of gold. A common thread we find among some of our friends is the one that ties them to the idea that everything good, active, and positive in their life is in their past. That wet blanket can destroy any feeling of purpose, or meaning, or forward motion in one's present life. Weren't you intrigued by the studies that showed that a sense of purpose can protect our mind from fading too early, that it can help prevent disabilities and even help lengthen our life? If our life seems to have some meaning, or we are able to feel we are contributing something, our life will seem richer until the end.

Much of this sense of purpose, or meaningfulness, must come from within, of course, but we all know that we do better in an encouraging environment. I never knew I could write until I was well into my fifties and a professor read a paper of mine and said, "You should try to get this published." No one had ever encouraged me before that time. Now I grant you, it might be a case of me being extremely simpleminded, but I like to think that it was the impetus I needed and the nurturing environment that made me look at myself a little differently, a little more positively. As a teacher, I always tried to remember that a positive comment here and there to one's students can reap rewards in the future that we may never know about.

I know I have mentioned it before, but it has been a concern of mine: I have had more than one person here tell me they wished they were dead. Life seems to have no more meaning for these souls, and they don't understand why God doesn't take them. Usually, but not always, they are those who keep to themselves. Which makes me wonder: which comes first, the isolation and lack of friendships, or the depression and wish to see the end of life? Occasionally it appears to result from family resentments, which gives credence to the research that shows that strong family ties are good for all of us. Anger over a perceived lack of attention from children, or a feeling of having been ignored in family plans, can create downer feelings, even though the cause of such feelings may be self-imposed or unjustified. In other cases, if one's past life seemed to be the source of importance and the reason to live, retirement at the end of one's tasks as an adult, as a parent, or as a successful businessperson can leave a void that is hard to fill.

When I encountered my first severely depressed person at Planet X who did not want to live, I really didn't know what to say, so I simply said, "Well, there must be some reason you're still here. Have you figured out what that reason is?" This seemed to make that person stop and think. I now follow with a suggestion that they decide why they are still alive. Consider: At our time of life (the average here is eighty-three), so many of our cohorts have already passed on. Those of us here may well ask ourselves: Why am I still here? What should I expect of myself? What can I do with this Brigadoon time?

Another dismal negative encountered in a communal setting is the person or persons who are so unhappy and bitter that they want others to be just as miserable. I think it's possible that they live in a residence with others just so they have someone to hurt: hurtful comments to servers at meals, and unkind, unsigned notes to other residents by a very few persons are a disturbing part of communal life.

I am convinced that when people feel that life is over, or are hurtful toward others, they are crying out for help, and I would like the professionals who are hired by Corporate to single them out and work with these people as part of their management job. Our reaction in America is often to simply say, "Well, if they don't want to be friendly …" or "If they don't like it, they should leave." Or in the case of the notes, "Well, what can you do?" If the professionals in senior care facilities would take more time to work individually with those who are depressed, I think that would be such a valuable service.

Recently management held a meeting to inform us of the therapy and help available to us. I found that we can get physical, occupational, and speech therapy, and help with such things as bathing, food delivery, medicine supervision, and even hospice care—everything at a price—but no real psychological help is available.

If one can see the problem, it is relatively easy to get help. But if depression or anger or paranoia are eating away at one's mind, it is not always addressed. Part of this is, of course, due to the lack of support from our insurance companies or Medicare. We must also remember that mental health treatment is not a favorite topic in America. Too many unhappy persons of all ages are currently walking the streets and sleeping under bridges. In America!

Obviously, this would be the place to put one's professionalism and psychology degree to work. It takes time, however, and a willingness to really get to know the seniors under one's care. It also requires investing in others. *These are some of the hurts that could be abetted by a person-centered residence for the elderly.* I'm not sure how mental health issues are currently being handled in assisted living or long-term care facilities, but in an independent living facility like we are in, such issues get little attention. What is the refrain we always hear when we disclose a problem? "This is independent living. There are no guidelines for us to follow."

I can almost see Corporate shrugging its shoulders and saying, "What can we do?" I wonder if as a society we have become too prone to believe that we should not interfere in another's private life. What if the person is crying out for help but no one answers because, "Oh well. It's their choice." Is it? Must everything be up to the individual? Is there no group responsibility for each member? What is the purpose of a government, then? What is the purpose of a residence for seniors? Is our present home only a holding pen for old people? As my cynical son said yesterday: "Solutions for warehousing." I don't think anyone would agree to that; no family would like to think that it is a place, a shelf, for the elderly to simply act out their depression, pain, and anger, and remain lonely.

Let me suggest private sessions or even group sessions with all residents, geared toward helping each one find a purpose or interest in his or her present life. It would take someone with some experience and training in group psychology, but surely, if Corporate is hiring qualified persons, there must be someone among the staff who could take on this job. Would that be so hard to do? Instead of the generalities, which we often get from Corporate, this would be a solid, practical project that would accomplish a real goal. With little effort, a friend and I have several residents involved in a writing group and are planning a possible literary magazine that we would publish every six months or so. Sometimes, you just have to ask and suggest.

We at Planet X are surrounded by examples of elders who exude purpose, and, as mentioned, we see others on the opposite track—those who, to the casual eye, appear to have dropped the word *purpose* from their vocabulary. I must introduce you to a good example of the first kind of person. I have grown quite fond of some of the older elders who live here. Recently, I walked into the library and there was E. She looked up at me with her bright, alert smile, and I was instantly intrigued. E. has already celebrated her 101st birthday, and yet I can't believe the warm, confident attitude that surrounds her. Whatever it is that she has, I want it.

I asked E. if I could interview her for *Shelved,* and she readily agreed. I sat near her, thinking she was probably hard of hearing, but no, she heard every word I said. It is so hard to believe that she was born in 1916!

"E.," I asked, "have you ever considered what your purpose was in life?"

She thought for a minute, then answered, "I was very poor as a child, and I decided I never wanted to be poor again. Oh, and I wanted to be a mother more than anything." (Practical and realistic, that's my friend.)

"Did you become a mother?"

"Oh, yes. I got married when I was twenty-nine to a man I divorced twenty-three years later, and we had two daughters. They still live close by."

This led me to another question: "So why did you leave him?"

"I honestly don't think I should have married him in the first place. I had a fine nursing career, and I think part of the reason I did marry him was to have children."

I realized then I was talking to a woman who knew what she wanted.

"Why did you wait for twenty-three years to divorce him?" I asked.

"Well, I didn't want it to affect the girls. So I waited till they were all grown and on their own." (Practical and considerate, that's my friend.)

"Have you ever been sorry you divorced him?"

Her answer surprised me: "Never! I began to live. I traveled. I enjoyed every minute of my life from then on. I did all the things I had wanted to do."

Again, a woman who knew what she wanted, I thought.

"So what do you think has led to your long life?"

"Well, you know, my mother was long-lived. I don't think she was particularly happy, but she had a real drive in her, and I think I've led a moderate life. I still walk, take yoga class, don't overeat, and I drink plenty of water." She smiled and added, "And I have a glass of wine two or three times a week."

"What advice do you have for younger people to help them prepare for old age?"

"It helps to be moderate in most things and keep busy. I do enjoy my reading and walking. Oh, and I love movies and the theater."

"What do you enjoy the most today?"

"I love to see and do things with my two daughters, my two grandsons, and my grandnephew, along with my five great-grandchildren."

I thanked E. and told her how much I admired her life.

"Well, you know, I'm ready to go. After all, think about it. I've lived one hundred years!"

E. is a dear. She has a friend to watch TV with, or occasionally sit on the bench outside in the evening hour. One evening I saw him put his arm lovingly around her shoulders, perhaps shielding her from the evening chill. They have their meals together and look after one another. I see the sparkle in E.'s eye and know that life for her looks to be very good. She deserves it. I find it hard to believe that she was sixteen when I was born.

Thinking about E. after I left, I realized she had some of the behaviors and conditions that research is saying can lead to a long life: her mother was long-lived, she's close to her family, she exercises, and she has a purpose in life, a little wine each week, sociability, and a joy of doing and being. This may make for longevity, but it also makes for an interesting individual. I sincerely hoped that day that I had made a new friend. And I had. What a delight she is! She may be ready to go, but I am not ready to lose her. As I walked away that day, I wondered how many residents or staff had sat down with E. to hear about her life. Like those of so many residents with whom I live, her life story is to be prized.

Looking back at our interview, I was struck by something that stood out: E. led her life and did not let her life lead her. Add to that the optimistic attitude of a woman who wanted to travel and enjoy her life. Positives all around and a life lived forward. What's not to like? What's not to admire?

Purpose can also be seen in the love between an aging couple. We have a fair share of couples at Planet X who, like us, moved here because one of the pair needed more help. It is common for us to see one member of the marriage caring for the other. We all age at different rates. "For better or worse" acted itself out regularly between two elderly lovers. J. and R. recently appeared in the dining room and our attention was drawn to them by the gentle care R. gave to his aging bride. J. was R.'s tiny, quiet, very slight companion confined to a wheelchair. She had a striking smile. R. was J.'s quiet, well-groomed husband who patiently and gently pushed her wheelchair to the table and tenderly lifted her into her seat. Like others here, this was obviously a man devoted to caring for his first love. She sat quietly while he placed the large napkin on her chest and fastened it around her neck, and then he sat.

Their story is lovely, and I only wish I knew more. As I recall, they began dating when they were very young when she asked him to a dance, and now, so many years later, they are still dancing in their behavior toward one another. Yes, this is one of those sad stories. J. became ill and went to the hospital for care, and when it was time to take her to rehab, R. brought her home to be with him. J. died yesterday and the staff and their friends are sharing the grief. Romeo is still here, but Juliet has gone on.

Have you ever noticed that there are some persons who have a light in their eye? I remember years ago meeting someone who had this light and I thought, "I want some of what she has." Often that light is there because they have found a reason to live, or have found someone to help, or they are doing something that makes them feel capable, or happy, or real, or close to God. If we were speaking religiously we might say they have seen the light. For our purposes here, let us say that those I have met who have that light have a mission, a goal, a purpose, or even a joy that we might all like to have. E. has that light, and, now that I think about it, several of my friends have that light. I will leave this up to the reader to decide why it is there.

I have also seen that light die, and it is very disappointing and sad. Someone I met the day we moved here appeared to live with such a purpose, but was not always doing other things that might extend his days. He said he wanted to live to 104 and be shot by a jealous husband, and we all laughed. But he lost his drive, his purpose, due to his health, and his lack of discipline in eating and drinking his life away. His own failings did nothing to allow him to live to 104. He couldn't give up the things that were killing him. Toward the end, his life seemed to have no attraction beyond his vices. By about two weeks before his death, I no longer saw any light in his eyes … only resignation. "I don't feel like this is home anymore," my friend said. Instead of 104, he soon died at 83.

A reader of an early draft of *Shelved* asked, "Can living at a place like Planet X help people find a purpose, a reason for their lives?" I think the answer is yes. Being around others who are motivated and participating in activities that stir that feeling of excitement within can make almost anyone find resolve. During an early chat, a new resident mentioned that his son had moved him here when he found his father was eating, sleeping, and living in one room in his house. I can't tell you what a change there was in the father after he moved to Planet X: tap dancing classes, happy hour friendships, and just sitting in the sun and chatting with friends. What a change in a human life. When I try to analyze why this happens, the answer seems rather simple: opportunity. It is fairly easy to interact and grow rich here from our contact with others. When faced with activities that strengthen the body, the mind, and the heart, this is how we deepen our self.

We have an excellent program planning team at Planet X, and there are endless opportunities to visit area points of interest, dine out, sightsee, and just go and do. Entertainments abound. This team generates great enthusiasm here with talent shows, art exhibits, special occasion dinners, and games galore. If we wished to make the researchers happy, we would probably need to emphasize more programs that open avenues to second chances, creative ideas, and volunteer opportunities, but I see these coming. I wager that more will be available as more residents request them. If we indicate a need on the survey they pass out each year, a way will be found. It is obvious that our program planning team cares about what we think and what we need.

Residents are encouraged to start their own classes or groups of interest. I'm thinking of D., who came with a dance background and is now teaching a tap-dancing class to a dedicated group of learners. They carry their tap shoes with pride and are planning a demonstration for our entertainment. The teacher appears to be blooming because she is doing something that captures her passion.

I was reading a book recently called *Lab Girl* by Hope Jahren. In it she talks about how her involvement in her lab captivates her, causing her to forget all else—about how she is completely absorbed by her passion for the work she is doing. In those hours she is completely fulfilled. This is the feeling I get when I write. Time escapes me and I forget my age, any problems I have with my health, my husband's issues, and feelings of loneliness or depression that might have been creeping up on me.

We need our passions. If we don't have one we need to invent one. There is P., who sculpts outdoors two days a week and has started a well-attended support group for women. It's amazing how popular this group is, and it shows that most of us are needy and unsure about how to grow old successfully. Through the exchange of ideas, we grow deeper in our own lives by getting to know how others are doing it. Yes, Dr. Vaillant, once again, we can't tickle ourselves.

However, one does not have to attend a class or group to feel needed and of worth. A purpose is fulfilled in life when one friend visits a friend in need, or takes it upon themselves to talk to and sit at a meal with newer residents. There is a purposeful action when we volunteer our time during elections or in the local action center to help the poor. Volunteers are needed at the Alzheimer's Association and so many other organizations. One of my favorite friends volunteers two days a week to help a local veterinarian. She loves animals and animals love her, and she goes home much richer than when she left early that morning. Another worked for a time at Walmart, greeting customers and passing out carts. A few are still doing bookkeeping for friends or relatives and keeping a hand in a career they loved, and there are residents who give time to the local action center.

Every day I see residents finding a sense of being needed right here at Planet X: helping wheel others to meals, calling friends to be sure they're OK, taking someone to the doctor, and on and on. We don't have to look far to find a reason to feel worthwhile; it is right there in front of our eyes.

The negative vibes emanating from some elders who find no possible thing to interest them are harmful to themselves and even more so to those who come in contact with them. Negativity is destructive, and it is catching. It is depressing to be near an old friend who insists on sitting on the couch and watching TV all day. He has nothing to talk about, with the exception, perhaps, of old TV shows and movies of the 1930s and 1940s, and he resists all attempts to get him involved, with the result that his body weakens every day and his brain atrophies. What a loss. What a shame. What could possibly cause such a downward turn? I think he lost his will to live years ago when he could no longer play the sport he loved. Today he could not play any sport. He can barely get into a car. How can we help someone find alternative interests when they seem to prefer closing the shell and waiting to die? I wish I had the answer to this question. I think we all do.

Let me give you an example of someone who is the opposite of what I just described. A program director brought G. into our knitting group a few years back when I was volunteering at another senior home. G. said she wanted to knit a sweater, yet looking at her, I doubted that she would be able to knit anything. G. had recently had a serious stroke, I mean serious, and her right hand was severely twisted and crippled. She managed to wheel herself to class with a great deal of effort and realistically said that, although she wanted to knit a sweater, perhaps it would be better to start with a scarf. I agreed, although I doubted she would even be able to do a simple knit stitch. We provided her with some yarn and needles and got her started. To my astonishment, with willpower she dug from somewhere deep within and a ton of determination, G. used that twisted hand to knit, stitch by painful stitch, until she finished that scarf.

No sooner was the scarf finished, but she had someone take her to the knit shop. Before we knew it, she arrived at class with a pattern and yarn for a sweater. Again, stitch by twisted stitch she patiently worked at that sweater until (need I tell you?) it was complete. When I left that group, she was on her second sweater, patiently proving that she was still a person deserving attention.

No one could look at G. and think she was only a damaged object. The will to live and succeed was engraved on her DNA.

Occasionally we discover a friend who seems to epitomize one's idea of a successful outlook and view of life. He or she would be the dream, the Exhibit A, of almost all the research studies I have read. Such is my friend H. I met H. while facilitating this same group of knitters in a local senior residence. She came up to me, put her hand gently on my wrist, and said, "I just love this yarn you found for me. It makes me smile—such a beautiful color." It was just a touch, but it was enough to make me smile and feel connected to her. I judged H. to be in her early nineties at the time. Her hearing was terrible, her hair was thin and gray, and she fell easily and slept poorly, but she was one of the most beautiful and happiest persons I have ever known.

Why is it that some of us, when we reach old age, silently throw away our dancing slippers and fold ourselves into our lap robes? What I saw with H. was a woman who had lost a husband, become unable to care for herself and her home, and received only an occasional visit from her son at this place which was now her home away from home.

She *was* happy, but what had she to be happy about? Not much, we could say. But unlike those who chase happiness in life, only to realize later that happiness is a side issue and is only found within and is a part-time friend, H. knew that all along. She was wise enough to know that joy is in the day, in the moment, in the wind, and in the outlook. She had long ago learned that life's joy is not found all alone on a shelf in a box when everything moves as we wish it to. And it does not come just because we demand it, cry about it, or pout if we don't see it in our lives. Chase happiness if you will, but you will not find it in any singularly impressive place. Nor must we consider it in the past tense. Happiness *is,* in every day's most common events.

H. constantly rewarded us with her words of happiness: "I'm so enjoying that wonderful three-volume biography of Teddy Roosevelt," she would tell us. When I inquired about her recent fall, she replied, "Yes, I fell and skidded all the way down the hall on my face and on my shoulder. You should have seen it. But I was OK. I knew I hadn't broken any bones."

Quickly her attention would return to the now: "I want to make a little shrug to wear at night when I read in bed, and I want it to be an elegant color and a very simple style, because that's me. I'm not very fancy. Oh yes, by the way, I'm so delighted. My friend is taking me to the mall, and I just know I'll find all sorts of nice things that I would like to buy."

On other occasions she would advise, "Oh, don't fret about the young. Give them a chance." When we saw H. enter the room, we automatically smiled; we knew that we would be better for having that hour with her wisdom and calming spirit. Happiness was not a *was* for H. She took care of life and let happiness take care of itself.

Moderation. Small helpings. Sample a little bit of everything. These are the secrets of happiness and good health.

—JULIA CHILD

I have mentioned it before, but I can't emphasize enough how important close family ties are for those in our age group. Research shows it and observation confirms it. It's very hard on those who have families who have mentally, and perhaps physically, shelved them, seeing them only now and then, perhaps just on a birthday or holiday. I really do not think families realize that this familial distancing can be very hard on elderly health. Emotionally we suffer when we're seen only when a grandchild needs money, or when we sense that visits are only a duty, not a pleasure. I know a gentleman here who seems glued to his chair in the lounge on ordinary days. He is often found napping and seldom notices anything that is happening in the world around him. Yet, given a visit from his daughter, the clothes change, the step quickens, and his eyes light up. I wonder if she knows how important she is to this old guy.

Yesterday I sat in the lobby drinking a cup of hot chocolate with a new friend. Since I didn't know too much about her, I asked her how she liked our state. (She had recently moved here.) "Well," she replied, "I thought when I moved here I would see my son a lot more, but that hasn't been the case. He's busy and so is his wife, so they seldom come over." It is difficult for younger persons to understand that when someone has given up their car, making contact is often a difficult thing for them. The younger members of a family sometimes must make the first move.

I remember when my mother was my age, and I regret that I, too, may not have been with her as much as I wish that others would be with me today. It is not the same when we are the elder. Age shows us the wisdom of loving those who have loved us. But then there is S. His two daughters are here so often, smiles on their faces, kidding and laughing with him. Perhaps they learned that from him, for even after a stroke and with serious health problems, that white-haired old man radiates a remarkable amount of joy.

Family love is the place for little loves. M.'s son comes to help get her smartphone operating. L.'s daughter fixes lamb chops on a Sunday during the football games. My own children are there when I need them and keep a close watch on us. I am so fortunate to have a daughter who is there when I call to ask her opinion on my writing—"Should I say it this way or that way?"—and a son who helps me fix my phone and computer, and is always standing tall on the instances when Dad or I end up in the emergency ward. That means so much. It may not sound comforting, but on one such occasion my son entered the ER, walked over to me, and said, "Well, I see you still don't have a tag on your toe." Believe it or not, as bad as I felt, I had to laugh.

My daughter observed that it is often hard for older folks to solve their problems alone, and I agree. Health issues can confound us, technical issues are not our forte, and sometimes we all need companionship, and just to know that our families care whether we live or die.

As I get to know Planet X friends better, I see how family dynamics can play a very large part in our happiness. Today, a friend was extremely depressed by an argument with a daughter. We listened, and as her friends we reminded her of the research that shows that, at our age, friends are even more important to us than family. Not that family isn't important. It most certainly is. But families need to live their lives, and our friends are there for us and understand the place in life that we are in at present. Our friend smiled and thanked us for being there, and I was, once again, pleased that we have gone beyond the superficial friendships that I had felt here in our first few months. Yes, we need our friends, and if we don't know them through thick and thin, how can we say we know them at all?

The more I see of the elder generation and the wealth of creativity and wisdom therein, the more I envy the corporate owners of Planet X, who have the pleasure of having such a great group of residents to assist. I'm not sure they are even aware of this, however. The staff is, I believe, but Corporate? I doubt it. We have so many of the Greatest Generation still among us. Purple Heart, Silver Star, and Medal of Honor are some of the awards that were given to several of the old guys with canes that you see here today. We have a gentleman who worked on the first A bomb and one who was in command of some of the moon missions. Yes, I really do hope they realize how much the old people they are caring for have done for our country and for our culture.

But let us discuss us in general: It is true that in *The Gift of Years* Joan Chittister sees some of us as grumpy and depressed, but Dr. Laura Carstensen, professor at Stanford University and director of the Stanford Center on Longevity, supports the idea that although the emotional dimensions of old age are vast and little understood, as the body ages as it is programmed to do, it appears that emotional stability thrives.[3] I'm not sure if I would call it stability—perhaps *flexibility* is a better word—and yet, even that does not quite fit our emotional place when we are eighty.

Older persons are more able to experience poignancy, Dr. Carstensen says.[4] That is, they can experience both positive and negative emotions at the same time. Possibly this is one reason some of us can see more sides to questions and to feel deeply down into our heart of hearts. Experience speaks to us, reminding us of both the happy and the not so happy memories of past loves, past friendships, and, yes, of our present time in space. I find I can laugh with my failing friend about the memories we share of when our children were young, and I cry easily when I see her suffering today. The poets can always say it better than I:

Go down to your deep old heart, woman, and lose sight of
    yourself.
And lose sight of me, the me whom you turbulently loved.

Let us lose sight of ourselves, and break the mirrors.
For the fierce curve of our lives is moving again to the depths
out of sight, in the deep dark living heart.
(D. H. Lawrence, from "Know Deeply, Know Thyself
More Deeply")

Now, with a bit of time and learning behind me, I thought of my heedless first thoughts about our new home. I was affected by what I saw—walkers, wheelchairs, white hair, and some bodies bent with age—and hadn't bothered to look deeply into the thoughts and determination of those around me. I was considering only myself and the inner disconnect I was feeling. As so often in my life, I judged too soon. My vision was dull. I was reacting to the negative image of old age that I had accused other Americans of holding. I didn't stop to ask who those around me loved, and who loved them. I had not taken time to see the wisdom that lay beneath each gray head. Like most of society, I had judged too quickly. It is so easy to do, but it is a practice that costs us greatly. And it is costing places like Planet X greatly when they, too, are not looking deeply enough at those they profess to serve.

Gradually I began to see the beautiful heart that so many of these now cherished friends possess. This morning a group met to discuss dreams, meditation, and divinity. The youngish leader kept us for a moment after our ending meditation with the statement, "I am so amazed at the wisdom in this group." Au contraire. We are not unusual. We are just old and experienced, and perhaps this has made us a tad wise. She sees something deeper within us—the effort we are putting into the understanding and the mindfulness of our lives. This is the wisdom Erikson wrote about.

Have we always been so wise? I find myself shaking my head no. Experience and our years have given us a depth we may not even know we have. Was I as wise before I moved to Planet X? No, I wasn't. I have indeed gone deeper into my own life by seeing how others here are leading theirs. I am now so much more enthused about my old age because of what I have read and what I have learned through my interaction with others. I am more understanding, more open to ideas I might never have considered in the past, quicker to speak up and act when action seems to be needed. This planet has been good for me.

Although not perfect, Planet X is attempting to escape from the outdated, dreaded vision of an old folks' home and the cold-as-ice nursing homes from the past that we pray to avoid. What I have studied so far has piqued my interest in becoming an actor in actively searching and sharing ideas toward the creation of an even more successful residence for seniors. As I have told many here, Planet X has the attractive structure, the location (a wooded acreage), and for the most part the staff that could be developed into a really excellent example of a forward-reaching place in which seniors may live happily and intelligently. It just needs tweaking.

Let me hasten to add that, although I may be critical of some of the corporate ideas, I realize their job isn't easy (even though Planet X is lucky to have such great people as us). Let me give you an example. The job I would not want to have, even for a million dollars, is to be in charge of the dining room. Every week we have Chef's Chat, which is the time when the chief chef introduces the menu for the following week and takes suggestions from the residents.

> *Chef:* "Well, hi, everyone. Here's the weekly menu for you to look over and ..."
>
> *Resident A:* (Interrupting) "The print's too small, I can't read it."
>
> *Chef:* "Oh, I'm sorry. We're going to read it out loud. Maybe that will be helpful."
>
> *Resident B:* "I don't see any liver and onions. I thought you said we were going to have liver and onions. I love liver and onions."
>
> *Chef:* "Ummm, well, we had liver and onions last week, and I didn't think we should have them every week, or ..."
>
> *Resident B:* "Why not? I like liver and onions."
>
> *Resident C:* "I can't stand liver and onions. Why do we have so much liver and onions? And all those red pepper flakes. My stomach just won't take red pepper flakes."
>
> *Chef:* "I'm sorry. I'll tell the cooks to go slow on the spices."
>
> *Resident D:* "I like spices!"

And so it goes. I think you get the picture. Meals in senior domiciles are of utmost importance. For some it is their major social outing of the day. They care where they sit, who they sit with, and what they are served, and they are vocal about what they are not getting. It really is almost impossible to please us all. Some don't try, but that doesn't work; some try too hard and are soon interviewing for a new job far away. The wise chef takes the concerns of residents very seriously and tries to hand us a dash of nutrition at the same time.

No, it is not an easy way to make a living, this trying to make seniors happy. However, one of the major factors that I believe makes further change difficult is not the seniors, nor the staff members who are trying hard to do what they have been hired to do, but the rigid corporate structure and the constant need for both compliance and profit. Corporate guidelines, designed to build consistency between a growing assortment of residences, is always aiming toward a certain outcome: the most benefit with the least expense. This is how corporations work.

Couple this with the fact that corporate boards are always aware of stock-holders peering over their shoulders, and the staff at the lowest level in the individual residence are aware of corporate heads examining what they are doing. This makes it hard to envision the kind of change we would like to see happening. What kind of change is that? My thought is that the residences would be geared to the individual instead of the institution, but we all know that the CEO would of course first ask, "How much will it cost?" Add to that the fact that management sees the good manager as "in control" and seldom feels free to share any of their decision-making power with the residents. All in all, the structures and any new philosophy have a chasm between them.

I had a long talk with my daughter and son today at lunch. I am fortunate in that they care whether we are content here, and yet they want us to be real-istic about what we can expect. I must be cognizant about the fact that any community residence is owned by someone, and in today's world that someone is usually a corporation. I need to remember, they said, that even though our country is a representative democracy, we can seldom expect anything other than an authoritarian type of association with corporate management. We have bought a service, my daughter reminded me, and the only thing to do if one does not like the service is to leave. There is a chance that the corporation might be open to more input from those living here if they feel a significant financial pinch, but otherwise the institution will act for its own benefit. Competition can be a prodding factor though, so as more and more senior facilities are built, and as boomers look for personal benefit in each of them, there is a possibility that significant change in how we care for our elders will somehow materialize. Is there currently an antagonistic attitude between residents and Corporate? I'm afraid, at times, yes there is, at least here at Planet X. It is there when we wish to have strawberry ice cream and are told that we can only have it at lunch, not dinner. It is there when we want a better light in the pool room and are told it wasn't on the approved budget. It is there whenever there is a denial of an individual need and we are told, "It's against corporate policy." We never know if that is true, because in some instances, as the staffer changes, the rule changes. This creates an atmosphere of serious mistrust. Add to that, when January comes and there is a hefty raise in our monthly rent, residents remem-ber all those choices they were refused in the previous year.

There is definitely room for improvement in the corporate understanding of what elders need during these last few years. Is it forthcoming? I don't know.

We receive brochures from Corporate telling us how elders act and what they need, and yet we know, as our Residents Council was told when we wished to survey residents regarding meals and dining room policies, "You are advisory only." Recently, after first being denied, we were allowed to conduct the survey, and yet most of us are sure that even though 65 percent of the residents voted for a certain change, it will not happen. Corporate rules.

Problems such as servers waiting on too many persons at one time could be solved by hiring another person, but that costs money. It appears that the ideas and suggestions designed by the seniors are too often overlooked and ignored. "We'll look into it." Never happens. When this happens it is difficult to feel that we have any worth other than our financial contribution.

Many in my children's generation do not see themselves living in similar places as Planet X. They are looking to places cooperatively owned, perhaps that will allow those living there to hire their own employees and develop their own lifestyle. In some areas, especially in eastern cities, there are more forward-thinking ideas, we are told.

Both now and in the future, care for the aged costs money, regardless of who pays for it. Cynically speaking, the color of old people care is green—very green. This is not hard to understand. It is so because old people require more care than young people do, and because the corporation wishes to keep the quality of service high, the resale value of their properties stellar, and the stockholders happy. This becomes increasingly expensive every year.

One reason for the continued increase is the yearly rise in what everything costs, and as the unemployment rate lowers, it is more difficult than ever to get and keep good help at the salaries most senior homes want to pay. This causes a serious turnover in the lower-paying jobs, making changing faces just an accepted part of life at places like Planet X.

Wouldn't it be nice to have the best cuts of beef and only the freshest vegetables? Of course, but compromises for the sake of the budget are constantly made. Does a dish take too many man-hours to complete? If so, it probably will not be served. Can we be served prime rib? Seldom.

Let us stress once again: professional care of the elderly is an industry, and make no mistake, it acts as an industry. And unfortunately in some instances, there is sham where we wish it wasn't. This is no surprise—there exists the possibility of sham in almost every aspect of almost every business. No one picks the worst aspects of any project to show to prospective buyers or renters:

possible new residents are shown all the finer points of the residence they tour, and sometimes promises are made verbally that cannot later be kept. This is just the way it is, and it requires prospective residents to be very careful and thorough in the questions they ask the marketing team of any senior residence they explore. You can be sure that if, when you move in, you are promised that dogs will not be allowed on that floor, and sometime later the only apartment available is on your floor and someone with a dog wants it, you will very likely have a dog as a neighbor.

Most residences have a front. I say this in the kindest way, and I am enjoying the benefits of Planet X's front, but *it is* designed to sell. The building itself was redone a few years ago to present a welcoming façade, and speaking from my own experience, it is quite effective with its large central stairway that spirals upward; greenery here and there; a boutique to the side with hot chocolate, fruit beverages, coffee, and tea; soft, inviting chairs and couches; and the delicious odor of popcorn wafting over all. I found the warm, comfortable library with books that are all up to date and a fireplace that is never lit especially appealing. Anyone might like to live here, and all of this is part of the standard tour for new prospects. It is all done with ease and a friendly smile and is quite effective.

However, be aware that real life happens here. People live and people die. I was not prepared for the turnover in residents that happens; some leaving to go to assisted living homes, others to long-term care residences, and some forever. There is also the occasional resident who leaves because he or she does not like the place, and the occasional resident who can no longer afford the tariff. I mentioned the friendships we develop here, but I have come to accept that some will leave us and too often we hear little of them from that point on.

Management wants to make it seem that all is well, and I really believe they would like it to be that way. The creation of a truly superior home for seniors is a very difficult task. There are ups and downs related to staffing and the disposition of the owners, as well as the personalities of those living here. Even more important is the philosophy of those who have designed the home—and don't forget the money. Philosophy and money. These two things determine how we will live at Planet X.

As senior care goes today, we at Planet X cannot complain too much. Life here, as I have said, is much better than life in senior housing just a few years ago. But I am speaking only of what I know: a rather expensive independent living home for seniors. And I will repeat, what keeps us here are (1) support is available when needed and (2) the friendships we have made both with residents and staff members. I am happy to not have the responsibility of our aging home, and I know I have friends and help here if needed.

> I learned this, at least, by my experiment: that if one advances confidently in the direction of his dreams, and endeavors to live the life which he has imagined, he will meet with a success unexpected in common hours.
>
> —HENRY DAVID THOREAU, *WALDEN*

> How vain it is to sit down to write when you have not stood up to live.
>
> —HENRY DAVID THOREAU, JOURNAL, AUGUST 19, 1851

EIGHT

The Employment of Being Old

As for old age, embrace and love it. It abounds with pleasure if you know how to use it. The gradually declining years are among the sweetest in a man's life, and I maintain that, even when they have reached the extreme limit, they have their pleasure still.

—Lucius Annaeus Seneca

We have talked about research, we have talked about Planet X, and we have talked about the scope of our life with others, but in the end, let us talk about the self. In the end we are all left with our simple soul, breathing, loving, and living our simple twilight life, and even with all the people around us, basically, even surrounded by loving family and friends, we ultimately live alone and we die alone. Leaving everything else behind, I want to consider in this chapter only one thing: what path, what personal decisions, what passions might my single soul undertake in these late years. How should I be employed when I am eighty-five?

It is not to be the kind of employment I might have considered when I was younger. It need not even be a job where I am *doing* anything. Rather, my direction for these years needs to be self-chosen and something that feels like a satisfying and culminating conclusion to my life, something that will leave loneliness and boredom behind and propel my old self into more wisdom about the nature of this thing I will call *Being*.

I have reached a point in my life that is beyond the minimum time expected, and it can even be considered a reward. If so, I may simply wish to sit back, try to enjoy life, and rock gently. Or if I see it as a time for reflection, I might close my eyes and figuratively remember the mountains I scaled, or sadly recall those I didn't. There is also the possibility that this may be the time in which I decide I want to discover a way to make amends for past faults, or, I might decide to spend this gift of time studying philosophy and unworldly thought so that I may peer more deeply into Being itself with the insight of age and years of experience.

Does this twilight melody, these wisps of a waning song, make me more reflective, or wiser? Can I now sense verities in life that were hidden from me at an earlier age? I am curious: What will I find if I search more deeply for wisdom concerning the mountains of my life? What has it whispered into my ear about Being and spirit and the sense of self that perhaps needs to be more clearly envisioned before being left for the next generation to remember? When I think on these things, I turn to the poetic and the sixth sense that we all recognize as we age—that sudden thought, those words that come unexpectedly and seem to help explain my purpose in this life more clearly, and the analogies that get to the gist of my life in a way I never thought possible. This is a treasured age.

It is obvious that what I do now will be eventually left to the ages, which makes it a good time to consider what impression I may leave. Let me consider a grandchild climbing onto my lap and asking, "Granny, what are some of the most important things I need to ponder in my life?" I guess I am asking, How do I teach my grandchildren to fly? Do I even know how to let my own spirit fly?

When I speak about meaning and life, let me explain what I mean. A memory comes to mind of the time when I was completely taken with an art exhibit my daughter and I attended. The exhibit celebrated the beauty and life in the quilts of the ladies of Gee's Bend, Alabama, a mostly black community south of Selma. It was a fascinating show of beauty, and I was so drawn to Mary Lee Bendolph's words displayed beside her quilt that I borrowed a pencil and copied them down: "I can't leave the spirit out. The spirit is all we had to lead and guide us back in that day, and it still is."

And it still is. Something whispers to me that what Mary Lee Bendolph considered to be of utmost importance in her life, and one of the greatest legacies we, any of us, can leave, is to foster the idea that "the sun is but a morning star," as Henry Thoreau claimed. What will we leave as a legacy if we leave the spirit out? Which path should we follow to open our eyes to the voluminous mysteries of the magic book of life?

> Don't believe what your eyes are telling you. All they show is limitation. Look with your understanding, find what you already know, and you will see the way to fly.
>
> —RICHARD BACH, *JONATHAN LIVINGSTON SEAGULL*

Jonathan Safran Foer, a young American writer and teacher, writes:

I'm grateful for anything that reminds me of what's possible in this life. Books can do that. Films can do that. Music can do that. School can do that. It's so easy however to allow one day to simply follow into the next, but every once in a while we encounter something that shows us that anything is possible, that dramatic change is possible, that something new can be made, that laughter can be shared.[1]

We all have a different way of determining what is beyond the sun, but for a beginning, let us start with the thought that what we see is only part of the enormity of what is and what can be. Foer's words simply show us avenues to follow in our search. It's not that I'm such a deep or philosophic person, but I have a real need to look beyond the lids of time, especially in this last third of my life, and I am fortunate enough to have been given the time to search and look and wonder.

My life here at Planet X is what I would call "semi-active." In the three-plus years we have lived here, I have found that we are lucky to live in such a complete senior home. It leaves us with time to use in a variety of pleasant ways. In writing memoirs I have felt a need to do as writer William Powers says in his book, *Hamlet's BlackBerry:* "Aim not widely, but look for depth."[2] Much of an average life causes all of us to wade in shallow waters, and as we deal with the things of a younger life, we splash about learning and doing what we see and what is before our eyes. But now is the Being part of our life—a time to tread in deeper depths if we so wish or feel the need.

I take Lucy out for a walk four times each day, and I would not trade this time for anything. It is perfect think time, Godspeed time, and, to paraphrase Mary Oliver from "The Summer Day," the time when I decide what I want to do with this precious life. It is as though Oliver and one of my favorite writers, Kerry Hardie, were walking hand in hand in their search for life's significance:

I know more or less
how to live through my life now.
But I want to know how to live what's left
With my eyes open and my hands open;
I want to stand at the door in the rain

listening, sniffing, gaping.
Fearful and joyous,
like an idiot before God.
(Kerry Hardie, from "What's Left")

Hardie is my absolute favorite Irish writer and one of my favorite writers in general. She has a way of thinking her way through her day-to-day life, making ordinary events seem special, giving meaning to the mundane and thought to the commonplace. I identify with Hardie's view of her daily life in which she at one and the same time is doing the daily "do," yet all the while ceaselessly considering and wondering and listening to the beat of life that pulses beneath all else.

Hardie causes me to wonder and helps me search for awe in the mundane. In my mind I see myself at that door in the rain, gaping, learning, wondering, sniffing, like an idiot before God and still trying, as Barack Obama suggested, to make sense of that rare quality, the audacity of hope. For me, this is how I long to see myself, using these last few moments before my magic book of life, my Brigadoon, closes and disappears into time. I might even fold my hands and send a word upward, hoping for comprehension beyond my own.

The message of Brigadoon is vague, and we are not sure why this magic existence appears and then disappears, any more than we understand why we have life and then we don't. Vaguely, love seems to have something to do with the magic of Brigadoon, and it may also be the most vital magic of life itself. I keep asking that question: Why? Why are some of us given more time than others to sing the last songs? Perhaps if I think deeply enough and love enough I will discover the "why" of my given time. Perhaps if I could just get some help:

Hey, You!
How should I address
the Almighty? Creator, Allah,
Higher Law, Jahweh, Oh Lord,
It all gets in my way of
talking to this someone, somewhere
who knows it all
and loves all.
Should I say, "It's me, Lord,"

or "Hi, remember me? Been
a while, hasn't it?"
Do I introduce myself, and
tell my geographical location,
religious affiliation or disaffiliation,
past sins and most assuredly
remind him of all my good
qualities? Can't hurt!
Or, do I say, simply and sanely,
"Hey you, I need all the help I can
get, and could you please,
please tell me
what I'm supposed to be doing?"
Amen.
—Sue
Oh, PS: Thanks for everything.

Ah, there's a thought. Could this particular idiot before God, with a little help, do something with this time so that I can then say, "Time, do your worst, for I have had today"? Is there some small thought or task that I can do today that will make me feel satisfied with the final me? When I was a small child, my mother would read to me the old English poem "Baby" by George MacDonald:

"Where did you come from, baby dear?"

And I would respond, "Out of the everywhere into the here." And we would hug.

This warm memory has lived lovingly in my mind, and has the spirit I am talking about. As my book opens to these final pages, I am here, living my simple life designed to live, to love, to do, to learn, and lastly, to Be. And when my magical book closes, I will take my unknowing but curious self back into everywhere. I want to be ready to leave. I want to feel that I am the best me that I can be, and that I have had the best understandings and perceptions I am capable of as I head off to parts unknown. I want to be pleased with my final self.

I don't know why I have been given the miracle of this time so that I may sing the last songs, but this idiot before God has a hunch that as I stand at the door of my life and gape in awe at the magnificence of God's creation, and look more deeply into the mystery of life, I may find one more tiny indication about what this life is all about. That's my audacity, that's my hope, and that's my dream.

I know I've told you that when my husband was suddenly very ill, I realized that I had opened my life's book to a page I knew nothing about. Growing old was written in what was to me an unexplored language, ignored by me as unimportant until then. Even helping my parents through their last years only partially prepared me for my own old age. I think I had unconsciously felt that this last act was not going to happen to me. I was like the lady in the pew who responded, "Who, me?" to the preacher's sermon about death and dying.

Suddenly, however, the possibility of life-ending illness had entered our lives, causing me to look more carefully at that final page in my book, and what I wanted to be the melody, the theme, of my life. It seems to me in my aging wisdom that at our advanced age we might be more content with these years if we have some inkling, some theme for the life we have lived.

In a strange way Planet X has afforded me the opportunity to share ideas with others as well as time to read and learn. One of my searches led me to *Creativity Matters: Arts and Aging in America,* which I talked a little about in chapter 2. In it the authors quote Dr. Gene Cohen, author of *The Creative Age: Awakening Human Potential in the Second Half of Life.* Dr. Cohen asserts that while problems certainly accompany aging, what has been denied is that there is *any* asset or strength or potential in old age. On the contrary, he says; the ultimate expression of this potential in old age is our creativity.[3] Think of it: to grow old, doing no harm, wishing to leave a positive legacy, *being creative.* When I read this, I knew that what I was seeing here at Planet X affirmed Dr. Cohen's words. It suddenly occurred to me that one of the most important tasks of those who profess to be in the elder business is to encourage us to find creative outlets. Herein is the meaning in our lives.

I have always been intrigued by the derivation of words: for example, *creative,* which means original or imaginative, derives from Latin words meaning to bring forth, or to bring to life. Albert Einstein is reported to have said, "Logic will get you from A to Z. Imagination will take you everywhere," and "Imagination is more important than knowledge. For knowledge is limited to all we now know and understand, while imagination embraces the entire world, and all there ever will be to know and understand." This is a view of creativity beyond coloring within the lines, and it was the thought that I needed to allow my heart and mind to open to thoughts and discernments that might take me beyond A to Z—to the imaginative, the creative.

Add to that the benefit Dr. Cohen shares: "Expressing ourselves creatively can actually improve health, both mentally and physically."[4] He explains that creativity reinforces connections between brain cells, strengthens morale, relieves sleep and mood disorders, increases vocabulary, gives us a positive outlook and sense of well-being, and even makes it easier to face adversity. All in all, creativity is one of life's ways of optimizing health and longevity.

Creativity: the ability to know and feel and think and write and do those things which one didn't have the time for earlier in life. *Creativity:* the ability to see the many avenues still available to us, avenues that may lead to broad expansions of possibilities of what life holds for us and what we can still add to life. Consider that the boundaries of practicality are no longer necessary for us at this time of our lives. This is the Land of Now. We are standing in the rain looking at our fading tomorrow. What does practical have to do with that? Let us not be practical. Let us learn to fly.

Dr. Cohen documents recent discoveries in neuroscience that radically challenge conventional assumptions about the aging brain. It is very true that the brain loses neurons as it ages. But it is not the number of neurons that determines intellectual capacity: it is the connections between neurons. These connections, known as dendrites, grow and develop when the brain is exposed to a rich, stimulating environment. Studies have also shown that between our early fifties and seventies the number and length of dendrites actually increase.[5]

If this is true, what dreams there are, what ideas may come. What memories can we reconsider and, perhaps, change our outlook or our reason for being? Creativity and choice, a way to optimize these latter years. There are so many highways and byways we did not travel in our practical, observable younger life. So many unplowed fields in this universe of ours, and a lifetime gives us only enough time to scratch the surface. We are all beginners in this thing called life.

Think of the paths we could walk together if we could stress the creative and work personally with the residents of Planet X. I had an exciting meeting with the regional executive director just a few hours ago. We spent some time dreaming of making Planet X the epitome of senior living by sponsoring groups and programs that foster the creative urge: carpentry, carving workshops, ceramics, writing groups, and groups that study the causes of depression and our feelings of uselessness that exist for some residents. If such activities are the only result from the publishing of *Shelved,* I will be happy. Of all the staff members here, I hesitate to criticize our program chair. She is so very creative herself and continues to come up with different ways to entertain us, but it is the creative that research recommends. We are seeing more programs geared to the creative, however, and since our program chair has a fine ear tuned to our welfare, I know we will see more in the future.

Leaders in the gerontology field in the 1970s conceived of the last years of life in terms of inevitable decline marred by disease and senility. The arts programs in senior centers and nursing homes in those years and following were no more than arts and crafts or sing-alongs intended to keep people busy. Today we have inherited some of this thinking, but more and more caregivers are beginning to understand that busy does not necessarily mean creative. Whenever I hear someone say, "Well, just keep them busy," I think of that. In those days, caregivers would wheel patients to arts and crafts activities fit for a five-year-old. The system was wrong. Elders, even if crippled, don't deserve to be treated like infants. Then, in 1975 Dr. Robert Neil Butler published *Why Survive? Being Old in America,* which linked Erik Erikson's theory of the life cycle to the process of aging.[6] Erikson, as we discussed in chapter 6, called the last stage of life Integrity vs. Despair. If I am led to see my life cycle as returning to the child, what can anyone expect of old age except depression?

Think of that choice for a minute. Dr. Butler saw reminiscence as central in this stage of life as a way to integrate one's whole existence—working out unresolved issues from one's past, present, and future—and he challenged gerontologists to actively nurture this process. One of the main aspects of his therapy was to recommend that elders be encouraged to write or meet in groups to recall events in their lives, or to listen to songs of their past and relate to them, or to share old photos with others and explain what they meant to them. So many mind-inspiring ways to live our final years and prepare ourselves for whatever the future holds.

Dr. Butler's research paved the way for senior homes to embrace activities of reminiscence: memoir writing, sharing, and unlimited creative activities. Some forward-thinking organizations slowly began to open the door to creative thinking. The Alzheimer's Association was way ahead of many places and persons designing programs for seniors. It has had a program called Memories in the Making for many years now. I remember it from the 1990s. Trained volunteers give workshops in art in Alzheimer's units, now called memory care facilities. The results were and are amazing. The cover of my first book (which was about Alzheimer's), *A Return Journey,* published in 2003 and reissued this year, was done by an Alzheimer's patient in the late 1990s. It is a picture of a lady, done in watercolor, who doesn't seem to know what to do with her hands. To me, the artist, who had dementia, knew what was happening to her. That picture broke my heart, but it shows me that the Alzheimer's Association was ahead of some others in recognizing the need to create, even by those with dementia. I highly recommend this organization and thank them for the help they gave me when Mother was ill.

Memories in the Making, which began in Colorado in 1994, has grown and is used in more than a hundred different communities. This is how progress moves: not in gigantic leaps ahead, but little by little, idea by idea. The Alzheimer's Association asserts that the program benefits residents in the following ways:

- "Improves self esteem
- Serves as an outlet for emotions
- Increase[s] attention span and focus
- Activates neurons
- Reduces isolation and provides opportunity to socialize
- Taps into pockets of memory that still exist
- Reconnects families"[7]

Today we are way beyond bingo and coloring books in our senior homes, and we've even added to activities of reminiscence. Memoir writing and genealogy are popular programs and more will probably be added if residents request them. Nevertheless, we are just beginning to expand our thinking about how to make old age a time of creativity. Another example of a current program is fitness walking, followed by a discussion of the music the walkers listened to on their headphones during the walk. Then there are book groups focused on music, biography, art, and philosophy, and I know of some senior residences that provide free music performances by faculty artists or students from various college campuses. We have had a different opera to watch every week.

In his book *L'âge de Créer,* French gerontologist René Laforestrie talks about a transformation that gradually takes place in us as we age, so that by the time we reach our old age, our life can be a vacuum that is filled with sadness, or nothing. He sees this as a choice: why not fill it with creativity, or love, or community service?[8] So let us continue our life's passion, or frolic off in a new direction of interest. Watch us dance, watch us paint, watch us write—just watch us and marvel that old bodies still have the glorious spirit of creative life within.

Dr. Laforestrie was one of the first to introduce art and other activities into the medical field. He calls the years of being old *l'âge de créer* ("the age of creating") and expresses a determination to reach elders, whom he believes society infantilizes. (*Infantilizes*—such a good word for what often happens to us.) He wishes to show that not only is creativity not lost in elders, but instead we have more to say than do youth. He sees a liberation in the perspective of the elderly that allows us to be independent.[9] At our age, we have no need for vanity. The designated work of a lifetime is done, and now is a time for our work to act in us as a liberating factor, freeing something powerful and new within ourselves. Now is a time to perform as an idiot before God.

Creativity is not limited to the arts. Creativity is designing a computer program, planting a garden, trying new recipes, conducting experiments, writing a poem, mapping genes, playing with children in the park or building a gingerbread house with kids. Creativity is making, inventing, producing—producing what? If we see nothing else of importance in creative activity, we must see that it leaves a legacy to others, and demonstrates the ability we have to find the love of life in our last days. Creativity is using and enjoying these last few moments till the very end in a desire to be the best we can be.

To go a step further, I was once interested in the work and words of Dr. Douglas Hofstadter, well-known professor of cognitive science who, when asked what thinking was all about, said this:

> The crux of the process is the act of stripping away the irrelevancies. I firmly believe that *gist* extraction, the ability to see to the core of the matter, is the key to analogy making—indeed to all intelligence.[10]

I ask myself, have I been given time to try to get to the gist of things: to strip away irrelevancies, or in some other way to get a glimpse of the core of life? We elders have the time now to use our minds, and research tells us that is a good and health-giving thing. The world is there before us, and we are past needing praise, so perhaps this is a time for us to use our resourceful minds to get to the gist of ourselves, to find gifts and abilities we did not know we had and to consider who we think we are. If not that, then perhaps it is a time to try things we have never experienced before. I have many current interests, but I need to focus and get to the gist of myself.

As I look back at my life, I see that during so much of it I was a daughter, a wife, a mother, a teacher. They were good times, but not necessarily *me* times. Plot-wise, the message for today is: Let nothing be postponed. Let me discover the gist of me—what I am capable of doing, thinking, being. Let us launch ourselves on the first wave that comes.

Various surveys show that elders want to feel productive, to do significant things, to contribute to society, and that many are quite physically active and like to be part of a group. This doesn't sound like how elders in America are currently viewed by the adult world, does it?

Before we go on, perhaps it is a good time to take a look at how we elders might be part of the problem. If we don't see ourselves as active, creative, and ready to be inventive, why should that be the view of others? Painter Vincent Van Gogh said, "There may be a great fire in our hearts, yet no one ever comes to warm himself at it, and the passers-by see only a wisp of smoke." When something (our attitude toward ourselves or our age, perhaps) interferes with that which gives meaning to our life, the need to find an outlet for our personal fire becomes paramount, or we can lose our enthusiasm and our influence. The word *enthusiasm* comes from the Greek *en theos* (in God). Without en theos, the spirit of life, the joy, is lost, and there is only a wisp of smoke for others to see ... and even more displeasing is that we ourselves may only feel as a wisp of smoke.

I spoke to a fellow resident yesterday about the possibility of telling her family story.

"No, no. I can't," she said. "I don't see well." I was not to be denied, however, and suggested she could tell her story on tape.

"No, no. I can't write." She shook her head, and I could see I was making her nervous so I stopped suggesting.

Some find it so easy to say no. Without that fire, there is only a wisp of smoke, but I feel that something will be lost when I think of the memories, the stories her children will not have because they will disappear with her.

I wonder whether some of us have ever taken the time to see if there is fire within. Perhaps we're afraid to look. I also wonder how many great ideas and memories have been lost over time because of fear. Unlike the bumblebee, which reportedly is too heavy to fly but does so anyway, we often are not encouraged to risk flight, nor do we have a view of ourselves as being capable of flight. I was trying to encourage a resident to come to our writing group, and she was flooding me with reasons not to. So I asked, "Are there no stories you'd like to tell your children and grandchildren?"

"Oh, my. Do I have stories!"

She then began to tell me her wonderful Western tales. She had stories, but not the will to sit down and write them out for her family. We will have to work with her.

Joy is found in those things that make us want to get up in the morning, and those who love us are happier seeing us with a fire in our eye than having to pick our emotional pieces off the ground. Granted, it is understandable that we should want to involve ourselves in something that is comfortable for us to do and enjoyable, but what if we withdraw so far that we don't see ourselves as capable of doing even simple things? If we have retreated this far, our fire can no longer draw others to our house. Ah, how sad it is to quit life because we negate our worth. Instead, let us look inside for the feistiness of old age, the time when we feel like saying, "Do it! Let others think what they will."

> Use the talent you possess: the woods would be very silent if no birds sang except those that sang best.
>
> —HENRY VAN DYKE

In a talk at a retirement community, Roger Landry, author of *Live Long, Die Short: A Guide to Authentic Health and Successful Aging,* told the audience:

> As a society, we marginalize older people. We pasturize them, is what I say, like putting a horse out to pasture. No. You want to move. Not jumping out of airplanes, but going for walks, taking the stairs instead of the elevator. Successful aging means minimizing your risk of disease and disability, and to do that, you've got to maintain your physical and cognitive function. You've got to be engaged in life.[11]

There is a purpose in taking care of our aging body: we have much to do and give before we die. We need to teach the world to fly. We are the mooring for those who follow. Our stories, thoughts, and creations can be the tools that allow our younger friends and family to glimpse the depth of thought that often takes a lifetime to learn. This is their anchorage. In these added years we can share our stories, our questions, and small thoughts, but let us avoid old judgments, old arguments, and tales of our past derring-do. We can help ourselves and perhaps those who follow to see the gist of life's meaning in the life we're now leading and what we are creating. Let us tell our loved ones what we're doing *now,* not live on past laurels.

Our competition is great, however: TV and electronic devices speak louder than the elder, who is the real repository of our culture. Stories of wise men and women, of true heroic action, of kindness to strangers; stories that help us sort out our morals—how do we determine good and evil?—these wise remembrances are replaced today by the easy, mind-numbing diversion offered by the entertainment industry. Add to that, too many of us, when we realize that we are part of the elderly generation, succumb to the stereotype: The Loss of Our Abilities. It is too easy to say we can't do this and we can't do that like we used to. Those around us usually try to sympathize and "try to make things easier." Yet even though such sympathy may be comforting, aren't we better off not looking for a release from an active life and creative thinking?

Let me tell you the story of a gentleman who loved golf above all else. In retirement he would spend four or five days a week on the course or in the clubhouse. But one day his shoulder became old and he was unable to play as he had before. Instead of playing less often or cutting back to nine holes, he gave his clubs away, accepting way too early the decrepit body of the old man. In two years he was using a cane and walking at a snail's pace—he who had made everyone run to catch up with him. His wife watched as daily he weakened and became more and more confused. We don't know what the final outcome may be, but … as we watch we cry, and we wait. What a waste, and how sad for those who love him.

Nothing must be postponed. Take time by the forelock. Now or never! You must live in the present, launch yourself on every wave, find your eternity in each moment … Take any other course, and life will be a succession of regrets.

—Henry David Thoreau, Journal, April 24, 1859

Often addressed as Grandma and Grandpa, and seen as nonessential to real life, we elders are regularly institutionalized in a vacuum of infantilizing and minimalizing, which can do its part to destroy whatever surviving gumption and creativity we have left. We may simply take a deep breath, sigh a bit, and adopt the stereotypes society has created for us while we slowly fade into the sunset. That's a choice. I, however, like to keep in mind this warning from Dr. Ellen J. Langer, professor of psychology at Harvard University and the author of *Mindfulness:* "Wherever you put the mind, the body will follow."[12]

As we age, part of our problem may be that we consider that we should be engaged in the same type of activities as an elder as we were as an adult under sixty-five. However, Dr. William Thomas, founder of the Eden Alternative program (discussed in chapter 6) and the author of *What Are Old People For? How Elders Will Save the World,* looks at these divisions in a different way, labeling our adult years as the *Doing years* and our elder years as the *Being years.* Dr. Thomas encourages oldsters to reach out beyond the rain and even beyond our known doorway, continuing to create, but in a different way than we did as an adult.[13]

According to Dr. Thomas, the adult years are when we are expected to *Do:* to make money, or keep house, or raise kids or ... the list of responsibilities we have from twenty-one to sixty-five is unlimited. He then explains what he means when he labels the elder years those during which we have the time to consider the *Being* of things. In other words, this is when we have time to look at the meaning of our lives. If we choose, the elder years are a time to search for depth and the emotional resonance of our soul—our Being.

When I consider Dr. Thoma ideas, I think that perhaps some of the depression we see in elders, some of the lack of confidence, is because many elders feel that since we are no longer able to *Do* the things we did earlier in life, there is nothing for us in this latter age. For some of us, it has been difficult to come to the day when we are no longer needed for Doing. Our age has been a fantastic Doing age—the age of World War II, nuclear energy, trips to the moon; the development of significant medical advances, phenomenal technical advances in aviation and communication and almost every avenue of visual life—and now the adult world doesn't need us. Doesn't need us? How sad, and yet, we have other responsibilities now, according to Dr. Thomas.

This thought caused me to consider a world without elders. What if today, persons over sixty-five were automatically terminated? What would this culture be without elders? I asked my daughter this question. She thought for a moment and said, "It would have no moorings." That says it all. Perfect word. She continued by telling me of entertaining a group recently and how she set the table with a cloth and silver from me, and china given her by her husband's mother. She told me that as she fingered these items, she thought of the history each represented. They were only things, but they took her back and connected her to her childhood.

I had to challenge her and suggested that these were just things, just stuff, material objects with little worth and less meaning. She countered by insisting that they gave her a sense of where she was in time and assured her that she, too, could contribute, just as each generation does. She felt secure in time, connected, and moored, just as a ship that travels the seas does its job and then returns home, sheltered and safe at harbor.

If we are the harbor, the mooring for those who follow us, what is our task at this late stage of our lives? We are no longer Doers. We may have lost our looks, and our general health suffers, all of which instruct us in humility and, if we aren't careful, depression. We can no longer look to the person we were as an adult but instead may have to search to find a message to live by in these final years. Again, I return to Dr. Thomas for some direction:

> To be is to create and sustain relationships with the invisible and intangible. *Being* yourself requires exploring who you were, who you are and who you wish to become. It is impossible for us to discover who we are, the Being of us, by Doing.[14]

The Being of life dwells in our thoughts, our intuition, and sometimes in our imagination, our creative spirit. An inward look is almost a necessity. I do not choose to disrespect those who have a great store of practical knowledge, but I cannot forget a quote by Ray Bradbury in *Fahrenheit 451*:

> Cram them full of non-combustible data, chock them so damned full of "facts" they feel stuffed, but absolutely "brilliant" with information. Then they'll feel they're thinking, they'll get a sense of motion without moving. And they'll be happy, because facts of that sort don't change. Don't give them any slippery stuff like philosophy or sociology to tie things up with. That way lies melancholy.

Thinking back on our lives, or considering the Being of our present life, can cause a sense of *melancholy,* or pensive sadness, which is a feeling we can deal with with more ease as we age. We can look more at the pensive than the sadness with the wisdom of age. Are we sad that the good days we remember are over? Yes, sometimes. But melancholy lives well with a word such as *poignancy,* which makes me think of the richness of life in general and even another favorite of mine, *serendipity,* in which we look for unexpected joys. All these words blend well with being eighty-five.

Hopefully, as we fondle some of the wild apples that have fallen in the corners of our life, thinking thoughts that may not be in the books, they will tell us something about who we are and why we are here. I have often wondered if the reason the choice pieces of life are so hard to find is that they are in the corners, the recesses, of life, and it takes the desire, or perhaps experience or even serendipity, to find them.

I am drawn to what the poet Stanley Kunitz is reported to have said: "We have to invent and reinvent who we are until we arrive at the self we can bear to live with and die with." This is part of our task of these later years, to search through the dregs of eighty-some years and find chips of hope, love, and eternity that will create the final *me.*

Now in this old age, we have the experience and depth to search for the meaning of our Being. This Being, or depth of life, that we search for is difficult to find during the Doing years, as Dr. Thomas tells us. We can ask someone to do something and see that it is or isn't done, but we cannot, with much success, ask someone to Be something. I cannot, by Doing, *do* love, but I can *be* loving. I can't do the relationship between husband and wife. It is just there, and it has a sense of Being. These are the intangibles and feelings involved in the Being of a person. Time, thought, and a deeper mindset are needed to encourage the Being in our soul. Love is a feeling, and feelings possess powers that are only dreamed of by tangible entities. These are the times to search for our Being, which is the gist of our personhood. Remember what Dr. Vaillant said of the Harvard research: the most important thing in our lives is love—full stop.

We can, at our age, deepen our Being with what we sense but cannot always see. We can search our emotions and feelings and share what we find through our creative efforts. Creativity is the pathway to finding this sense of Being. As Dr. Thomas says, people who are close to death do not wish to have more time on the job. They are closer to the Being of life and need the love and closeness of friends and family. Recently a good friend died. And before his going, he expressed concern about being a burden to his family. Only by showing their love and holding him close could his family still his fears and help him to feel their concern.

As my book of life begins to fade, I want to consider the Being of me and my place in time. In *What Are Old People For,* Dr. Thomas says that "to *Be* is to create and sustain relationships with the invisible and the intangible" and that our life requires "a constant refashioning of who we are, where we are going, and what we want to be."[15]

It is this need to understand intensely that takes us to the deepest veins of life itself. We find depth and meaning in the Being part of ourselves. We can only make wise guesses about why we are given life, but it is in our Being moments that we can chew over the possibilities, be they religious, philosophic, spiritual, or scientific.

We are the fortunate; we who now have the time in which to explore the Being of ourselves and the universe. This is one reason I see for emphasizing the arts in these years. Feelings, emotions, and insights can often be best expressed through poetry or art or music. We can find meaning in this exploration and deepen the real significance of our senses. Yes, the search may be melancholy, but the results can add poignancy to our lives, leaving us with some serendipitous moments.

But simply to Be is not all Dr. Thomas challenges us to do. He also assigns us some tasks for our final years: (1) to work toward peace, (2) seek wisdom, and (3) be concerned for the creation of a legacy. Searching for peace in this troubled world is obviously a worthwhile goal. Conflict is senseless as we age. Actually, it's worthless for everyone. Physically, and even mentally, we are no longer ready for battles of any kind, and although it may seem like a sign of weakness, we no longer have to vie for prestige or even prove we are more successful than anyone else. This freedom allows us to take on the role of peacemaker. We no longer need to push our children or grandchildren into roles that we have preordained: let us tell them, Thomas advises, "Do your best," "Be happy," "Be proud of yourself." This is the gift we can give to an anxious world and to those we love.[16]

As a peacemaker, first I have to make peace with myself, and this is perhaps the hardest task of all. I must forgive myself for opportunities missed and mistakes made. *Peace.* Then, I can try to bind up any wounds in our family. All families have them. I think of my step-grandfather: when my grandmother died, he turned on my mother, accusing her of not taking care of her mother. Mother had spent months as a caregiver to Grandma and was grieving and exhausted at the time of his attack. How noble he would have been had he gathered my mother into his arms and said, "I know you did your best, and she loved you so very much." Instead, the family split, and never again did he see my mother. And my mother never forgot his words.

Yes, I believe it takes courage and wisdom to face the wounds of family life and set out to soothe them, putting anger and misunderstanding aside.

Old age hath yet his honor and his toil.
Death closes all; but something ere the end,
Some work of noble note may yet be done...
(LORD ALFRED TENNYSON, FROM "ULYSSES")

I overheard a conversation between a resident and a server at lunch today:

"What is there about potato salad that you don't understand?" the resident spat out.

"Sorry, I'll go get it."

"See that you do."

This is not a work of noble note suitable for our last days. It's shortsighted, dogmatic, and shows a lack of verbal ability to solve problems graciously, or peacefully. We don't need to start a full-fledged war to express a need.

Let us go beyond peace to see if there is any wisdom within our Being. Probably the most important task of our latter years is to discover what wisdom we have gained from all the years we've lived and the experiences we've been through. If you're like me, you hesitate to declare that you are wise. Wisdom hides in the Being and seldom in the Doing part of our existence, and it is highly undervalued by society as a whole. The TV program *Jeopardy* encodes us to think of wisdom as how many facts one can retain and spit out on command. Although playing Trivial Pursuit may strengthen the aging mind, a definition of wisdom in my Oxford dictionary is "the quality of having experience, knowledge, and good judgment." Facts alone do not necessarily make wisdom.

Another definition of wisdom says it consists of three key parts: cognition, reflection, and compassion. Sadly, the idea that elders have value, let alone wisdom, is highly suspect in a society that places so much importance on the answers to the questions what do you do? and what have you done for me? Currently, American society is more likely to speak of the elderly as grouchy, opinionated, and often a bit daft. Seldom do even we elders think of ourselves as wise.

By our age, we certainly are experienced, and we must have displayed some knowledge as we trundled through life. But it is good judgment, compassion, and the ability to reflect on our lives and find wisdom there that are now needed. However, instead of displaying wisdom, we often find that the younger generation listens to us with rolling eyes, if we insist on talking about our early years when we did blah, blah, blah. At such times we may be pampered with a smile and a nod, but we are not really taken seriously. Our captive audience may listen to us, and yet pity us because we have nothing current to discuss. Talking about our past is not considered sharing wisdom, and pity is something I do not want. Aside from pity, sometimes we get that "I'm nobody" feeling, which is the antithesis of feeling wise.

W. Somerset Maugham, in *Of Human Bondage,* writes of Philip Carey when he returns home to the parish where his aunt and uncle still live. Philip is nineteen and full of the steam of youth:

> Philip realised that they had done with life, these two quiet little people: they belonged to a past generation, and they were waiting there patiently, rather stupidly, for death; and he, in his vigour and his youth, thirsting for excitement and adventure, was appalled at the waste. They had done nothing, and when they went it would be just as if they had never been.

Philip saw no wisdom in these old people, only wasted lives spent building a cage of limited expectations—wake, eat, do their prescribed work, then to bed, only to repeat the process again and again—while they wait stupidly for death.

One wonders why anyone would allow themselves to fall into such a trap, and one also questions why we allow this version of our lives to be what younger persons often see instead of any wisdom we might imagine ourselves to have. It certainly isn't received as wisdom when our thoughts are preceded by "You oughta" coming before our supposedly wise advice. Another geezer comment that causes a youthful sigh is, "Now, when I was young …"

Let us not downplay our wisdom. Research shows that even though cognitive functioning slows as we age, speed isn't everything. A recent study in *Topics in Cognitive Science* points out that elders have much more information in their brains than younger persons, so retrieving it may take longer. Add to that, the quality of the information in the older brain is more nuanced: older people show "greater sensitivity to fine-grained differences," the study found.[17]

Wisdom lies somewhere in those thoughts that nibble at the blank puzzle of life itself. For example, a few years ago there was an eighty-six-year-old member of our knitting group whom I considered wise. She was very hard of hearing, but rather than complain about not hearing the conversation, she simply added a note of her own—a story, a thought, a question. I remember one time when I was being critical of my husband, she quietly suggested, "And you'll miss him when he's gone, won't you?" Not *but,* but *and.* And with that small word she had added her thought to what I said, and yet I did not feel criticized. She never said, "You oughta love him now, for you don't know how long you will be together."

I still remember the words of the grandmother of a friend: "Everything in life will make you bitter or better," she told us when we were about fifteen. I cannot count the number of times my mind has returned to those words, and I do believe they have helped me be more positive than I might have been without them. It is our task as parents and grandparents to help the next generation deal with a world full of confusion and anger, and to do it wisely—not by imposing our way of life upon them, but by empowering them to find wisdom in the ordinary events of their generation.

Long after my death, I hope my grandchildren will think of things I have told them, as I remember my own grandmother's patience, understanding, and wisdom, all made beautiful by her strong faith and her loving nature. I learned so much from her, and yet she never sat me down for a lecture. Grandma had only an eighth-grade education, but even today I can feel the love and strength she shared with me.

When I was about three years old, she let me go with her to the potato patch down in the Wabash River bottoms. She would give me a spoon and let me dig and discover the magic of what the earth could produce, and all I felt the whole time we were together was love. A few years ago I wrote this about my memories of Grandma:

WHAT I LEARNED FROM MY GRANDMA
Dig carefully, so as not to hurt.
Glory in the magic that life unfolds.
Live patiently,

in order to accept what is.
Love completely,
with concern for the giving more than
the receiving,
and trust that there is more to life
than what we see.

Sometimes it takes years before we learn to appreciate wisdom; so elders, tell your stories and they will be remembered, if not now, in years to come. Even today, more than eighty years later, I can still smell the damp soil in those river bottoms and feel the love when my grandmother would shield me with her flour-sack apron, while at the same time educating me about how to be useful and thoughtful.

My friend M. wrote the following to her granddaughters as they went away to college. In their own way, her words form a sound structure for the next generation of women to consider. M. has phrased the advice in humorous yet sound lingo for her youthful granddaughters to understand. It is one generation's wisdom being shared with the next generation in such a way that it doesn't sound like Granny ordering them to do something:

GRANDMA'S ADVICE
The most brilliant professor was once a teenage kid.
Be strong—don't let anything or anyone control you.
Being pretty is an asset, not a lifetime goal.
Males and females are different. They look different, they act different,
    they think different. Accept it, it's not going to change.
Choose friends who like you even when you have a runny nose and diarrhea.
Accept the fact that no one is perfect. How dull would that be?
If you like your roommate, you're lucky. If she likes you, she's smart.
Choose your girlfriends wisely and your boyfriends carefully.
Have fun, but if that's your sole reason for going to college, buy a surfboard
    and an airline ticket to San Diego.
Be nice to old people—they're just young people with wrinkles.

Wisdom is of the moment: a word, a gesture, a smile, or, in certain instances, the wisdom to stay silent. M. phrases her truth in such a reasonable, understandable way. We all have legacies to leave, but what you have learned and wish to pass on is probably far different from any knowledge or sense of being that I may have singled out. Like snowflakes, each message we send, each choice we make will fall on this or that branch, leaving our legacy behind. We may never know just where the words and thoughts we leave behind will land, or who will suddenly gain a new insight because of a fleeting moment we have shared. In my humble opinion, where we go with wisdom has no boundaries, and in most cases it defies definition, but it is limitless, profound, and as wide as our minds allow us to travel. At times we sense that wisdom can move us beyond A to Z. Let us not define wisdom or issue edicts that will limit understandings or insightfulness. Like all universals, these things are unbounded.

The final task we were given by Dr. Thomas was to think about what we want to leave as a legacy. Do you recall what Dr. George Vaillant of Harvard said? That if we haven't done something before, it is never too late; like opening an IRA, we can start leaving a legacy any old time. Think of all the people who have made great contributions well into their later years—for example, the artist Grandma Moses, Colonel Sanders, Peter Mark Roget, who wrote *Roget's Thesaurus* in his later years, and Norman Maclean, who wrote his first and only book published in his lifetime, *A River Runs through It and Other Stories,* at age seventy-four. I am not famous, but I had my first book published at seventy-one. No, it is never too late.

No one can leave the legacy that another leaves. If we are the security, the anchor, the wise ones of our society, then one of the main purposes of this time is to develop the wisdom of our life, to tell our stories, and to leave a legacy of purpose and love. Even if all we do is display some wisdom in a peaceful way, we will have left a legacy. Preaching is useless unless we walk our talk.

There may be a difference between the elder and the elderly, however. Age does not automatically bring wisdom that we can pass on to others. In the book *From Age-ing to Sage-ing: A Revolutionary Approach to Growing Older,* authors Zalman Schachter-Shalomi and Ronald S. Miller quote June Singer, a Jungian analyst:

> The elder differs significantly from the rather rigid, authoritarian picture that many of us have of the elderly. The conventional older person ... generally resists change, holds on to power tightfistedly, and frequently imposes his knowledge on others unsolicited. The elder, on the other hand, is flexible, unattached to outcomes, tolerant and patient, and willing to teach

when asked…. Such a person radiates an enormously beneficial influence by evoking the questing spirit in younger people.[18]

I love what Singer says: to evoke a questing spirit in those who follow. No better legacy could I leave than that those who follow would have a questing spirit—to ask, to seek, to question, and to continue this through their lifetime—and would that I had had some part in that.

In a recent chat my daughter shared with me that she had had a difference of opinion with a long-time friend and that she was hurting from some very contentious comments her friend made. Then she said, "But I remember what you told me about Grandpa. That when the neighbor had been angry, Grandpa said to Grandma, 'When they throw stones, you throw back bread.'" So wise, and Grandpa would have been very proud to think that his granddaughter—whom he had met only once when she was five months old—so many years later would cherish his words, his wisdom. This is a legacy, and it is the best kind of legacy. It is the gift of love.

No, we cannot impose our wisdom or our beliefs on others. Leaving a legacy is not a Doing activity. A legacy is often created without our knowledge. It is left in the corners of our life, among the dried leaves of words we may have uttered or love we may have shared—denied.

Live with skillful nonchalance and ceaseless concern.

—Prajnaparamita Sutra

Perhaps we will never know what legacy we have left, or to whom we have left it. Friend M. gave to her granddaughters great ideas wrapped in such a way that they could see their wisdom. Friend B. will leave a sense of humor to those who follow, not by telling them to have a sense of humor, but by sharing her uncomplaining and kindly way of life. Even with four joints replaced, she still can smile and make others smile. B. is like that. Using her walker, she trots herself to church, adult classes, writing groups, and multiple activities. She always has time for a smile, and took the time to write the following humorous story:

Since living at [Planet X], I take for granted that our environment is mostly handicap accessible. There are elevators so we don't have to climb stairs. There are grab bars in the bathrooms. With the exception of a few chairs in the lobby, most have arms and are easy to get out of. Not so in the real world. I recently visited my daughter-in-law and grandchildren at their new home. It's a lovely home but definitely not grandmother friendly.

To begin with, there are three cement steps with no railing leading to the front entrance, so I need a shoulder to lean on in order to enter the house. The bedrooms are on the second floor, so I have to climb the stairs. My grandson has kindly loaned me his bedroom, but his bed has drawers underneath and it is so high that I need a stepstool to climb into bed. The toilets are too low. Most of the chairs don't have arms, so I have trouble getting up. If I sit on the sofa, I sink in and need a hand up. The trouble is that when I sit down, I forget that I'm going to have to get up eventually.

Our church is remodeling the sanctuary, so services are held in the Fellowship Hall, where we sit on folding metal chairs. By the end of the hour my posterior is paralyzed. Getting up and down is so difficult that I usually just sit during the service. Yes, it's a relief to come home to [Planet X], where I feel comfortable, where life is geared to those of us who don't get around as well as we used to.

The legacies of both M. and B. are moorings for those who follow.

Looking, asking, finding, studying, sharing; alive, interesting, humorous, and using the powers we have left to the max. What a great gift this old age can be to ourselves and others if we wisely use our talents to create such tender legacies.

What can a legacy do? It may help others see life as bigger than an individual opinion. It may show those to come how to find a purpose beyond themselves and their wants and desires. It may describe how others feel. A legacy may show a depth of love, or, on the other hand, it can show anger, or hate. An inheritance left can be in stocks and bonds, but perhaps, more importantly, it could simply say: I hope life matters to you, and that I have helped you in some way.

Everyone must leave something behind when he dies, my grandfather said. A child or a book or a painting or a house or a wall built or a pair of shoes made. Or a garden planted. Something your hand touched some way so your soul has somewhere to go when you die, and when people look at that tree or that flower you planted, you're there.

It doesn't matter what you do, he said, so long as you change something from the way it was before you touched it into something that's like you after you take your hands away. The difference between the man who just cuts lawns and a real gardener is in the touching, he said. The lawn-cutter might just as well not have been there at all; the gardener will be there a lifetime.

—RAY BRADBURY, *FAHRENHEIT 451*

Ray Bradbury died just a few years ago, and the legacy he left is a mighty powerful one. Few have had a way with the English language that Bradbury possessed. Few have worked with his diligence and insight, or have taught lessons of peace and wisdom as he did. The gardener will be there a lifetime.

Yes, everyone leaves a legacy. Often elders fall into negative patterns because they see no future and have given up trying, without realizing they are creating a sad legacy they might not wish to leave if they took the time to reflect. At such a crossroads as old age presents, we can rest on past laurels and spend the remainder of our life rocking, watching TV, and sharing our aches and pains with one another and our relatives, resting on our society's inherited pessimistic stereotype about aging. We've earned it, we can say, just to sit and rest all day. Or we can expect our families to make us happy. That's another negative legacy.

We have a new resident here who was asked if she likes it here. "I hate it," she said. "My son made me come here, and I don't like it at all." When she has left this mortal coil, her son can honestly say, "I could never make her happy." But did he really try? Did she? What will her legacy be?

I remember the grandmother that I mentioned before with the fondest feelings I can muster. She was gentle and kind with a marvelous sense of humor, and she taught me love. I also remember my grandfather on the other side of the family. He was cruel and abusive to his wife, my other grandmother, and full of malicious comments whenever we visited. I want to choose my legacy carefully, because I *will* leave one, and I want it to be one I really want to leave.

A legacy is left when those left behind are wont to say, "Remember when …" and tell a story about something that we said or did. A legacy is left when someone sleeps under the quilt we made, or wears the sweater we knit. A legacy was left when someone I barely knew told me of my father's goodness and how much he admired his skillful handiwork. A legacy was left when I found my father's book collection and realized the expanse of his interests and knowledge. A legacy was left when I looked through the home décor magazine clippings my mother collected. I never could make a room have the aura of home as my mother could. My mother's legacy is there when I talk to people who knew her and they tell me how they remember her friendship. My kids also remember her awful bean soup, but this is a warm memory, as if it were the nectar of the gods. We laugh and remember.

Though small, these legacies warm my heart and bring my parents, gone for many years, closer to me. And bring a tear to my eye. Memories, memories—whether good or ... These are our legacies.

We have little way of knowing what will be remembered about us once we're gone, but to work for peace, to use our experience to teach us some insight and be aware that we are leaving a legacy must surely give our years some purpose, and will surely keep them from being wasted. These are the tasks of Being. Thank you, Dr. Thomas, for your excellent insight.

As the Pulitzer prizewinning poet Galway Kinnel said, "Everyone knows that human existence is incomplete. Among those who are especially troubled by this are those who turn to writing. Writing is a way of trying to understand the incompleteness and, if not to heal it, at least to get beyond whatever is merely baffling and oppressive about it." My own writing has led me to select a few projects I want to tackle over the next months or years. I agree with Mary Oliver, who says in the last line of her poem "When Death Comes," "I don't want to end up simply having visited this world." Hopefully, if time allows, I will find the self I'm willing to die with. In my remaining days, or weeks, or years, I want to:

1. Take time to appreciate the beauty of the world. I will take walks and see the wind in the trees, and count the different clouds in our skies. I will enjoy breathing and consider how good life really is and how lucky I am.
2. Look more deeply at the meaning of this life. Why am I here? I want to live mindfully, looking for hidden or even spiritual metaphors in the things of this world. The many lessons of nature are all around me every day of my life. Let me learn all that I can.
3. Read and seek out activities that will take me to the being part of my life that I can understand. I want to read books that make me ponder and even question.
4. Work to be humbler and to accept myself and others.

5. Practice the things of the spirit: religion, meditation, and the study of past spiritual leaders. I want to look inside myself to see who lives there.

6. Be there with friends when needed and be willing to share with friends as needed.

7. Find time for poetry. I yearn for poetry. I devour books of good poetry and even write bits of poetry myself. Stanley Kunitz said, "A poet needs to keep his wilderness alive inside him. To remain a poet after forty requires an awareness of your darkest Africa, that part of yourself that will never be tamed."

8. Henry Thoreau would encourage us to dwell in our wildness, to explore it and to connect ourselves to the poetry of nature and of nature's lessons.

9. Exercise and practice eating well so that I do not destroy the gift of my body sooner than necessary. I need to learn to deal better with stress, and perhaps a glass of wine at night wouldn't hurt.

10. Journal. Journaling helps me see the fractals of my life. It helps me view my life as a daily journey rather than a continual, often meaningless, trip. Through journaling we can see beyond the obvious and into the soft, gentle, spiritual side of ourselves.

11. Keep my friends and develop new ones. I love my family, but I need my friends.

12. Care about the things of this world. I found that I had gotten to the point where I didn't want to care who became president in 2017. Then I remembered a couple of lines from Mary Oliver's poem "What I Have Learned So Far": "the gospel of / light is the crossroads of—indolence, or action. // Be ignited, or be gone."

Personally, I can think of no better way to end this discussion than to remember the words of William Wordsworth from "Ode: Intimations of Immortality from Recollections of Early Childhood":

What though the radiance which was once so bright
Be now for ever taken from my sight,
Tho nothing can bring back the hour
Of splendour in the grass, of glory in the flower;
We will grieve not, rather find
Strength in what remains behind;

In the primal sympathy
Which having been must ever be;
In the soothing thoughts that spring
Out of human suffering;
In the faith that looks through death,
In years that bring the philosophic mind.

NINE

Last Times, Last Thoughts

> When we spend our lives waiting until we're perfect or bulletproof before we walk into the arena, we ultimately sacrifice relationships and opportunities that may not be recoverable. We squander our precious time, and we turn our backs on our gifts. Those unique contributions that only we can make. Perfect and bulletproof are seductive, but they don't exist in the human experience.
>
> —Brené Brown, *Daring Greatly*

At this later stage of my life, along with uncertainty lives more uncertainty. Aside from all the practical aspects of preparing to no longer be present, and at the same time show up, and as Brené Brown says, "let ourselves be seen," we can't help but wonder. We wonder a lot. Will we be able to "push to the end?"[1] And when we get there, what then?

Practically speaking, we have to be sure that our will and final papers are all in order, that we have a designated power of attorney, and we need to relay our last wishes to those we will leave behind. Most of us have no problem with taking care of these little details.

Then what? In our case we had to decide where to live and where to get help when and if we would need it. My biggest question was, do I have the *courage to be* and *do* and not let time slip away unused? It is so easy to do so. Our society and perhaps even we ourselves don't see our actions of any account. My second question was, do I have the strength, the ability, and the pluck to attempt any far-reaching, or even near-reaching goals? Some of the goals mentioned in chapter 7 seem mighty imposing to someone my age. Do I see myself as showing any wisdom when I am vulnerable and just plain old? And my biggest worries are whether I can deal with the day-to-day problems that a couple our age has to deal with and, when I have time to think about it, what legacy I will leave. And, and, and…! I wonder a lot.

Old people may be seen sitting around, ostensibly doing nothing, but perhaps they're not just sitting, but also wondering. Perhaps they're deep in thought, knitting the last threads of their lives together, hopefully into something that seems of some value. I don't wish to be particularly maudlin about all this, but so often we skip over the painful thoughts without dealing with them and it doesn't solve anything, it just buries them still deeper. There are times when these thoughts need to be pondered.

Obviously this is a time of reflection and meditation, but beneath my mind's chatter has to be the acceptance of the fact that my time here is only a footstep. Many footsteps have gone before me and many will come after, which leaves me, and each of us, with only a tiny toehold on the universe. I am content, however, that anything I may attempt today may have to be completed by another. This is the nature of things. We are all only a step in time.

Elders are realistic. We know that our time is about up, and that whatever we do in these years must be done fairly quickly, with a lot of luck and … with something more: courage. The title of one of Brené Brown's recent books, *Daring Greatly,* quoted at the beginning of this chapter, says it all: can I get past depression, loneliness, the illnesses, age, and doubt in my own abilities and still be willing to open myself to challenge and opportunity until the very end of my life? Maybe.

I have to remember, if I do not walk the walk and stand tall now, when will I? Fear, caution, and a feeling of ineptitude can cause me to squander this precious time. What a painful waste.

The wonder of something beyond ourselves is not limited to old age, but in these later days there are definitely last thoughts of something beyond ourselves: it is called *awe.* Albert Einstein describes it as the sensation of the mystical:

> The most beautiful and most profound emotion we can experience is the sensation of the mystical. It is the sower of all true science. He to whom this emotion is a stranger, who can no longer wonder and stand rapt in awe, is as good as dead. To know that what is impenetrable to us really exists, manifesting itself as the highest wisdom and the most radiant beauty, which our dull faculties can comprehend only in their primitive forms—this knowledge, this feeling is at the center of true religiousness.[2]

Einstein's spiritual faith is the subject of various interpretations, but let me pretend I wrote the above and take it as my own opinion. I'm not sure what Einstein's final beliefs were. I only know what he wrote.[3]

Philosopher Paul Tillich, in his book of the same title, calls the ability to live with this sense of awe "the courage to be." As I understand Tillich, he reasons that we need the *courage to be,* in spite of … in spite of doubt, in spite of our "dull faculties."[4] Uncertainty and awe are a part of life, both the scientist and the philosopher tell us, and in spite of not having any guarantee of something beyond ourselves, we live, we do, we ponder, but we go forward.

As a Christian existentialist, Tillich also saw the wonder that Einstein, the scientific genius, describes. Both were aware of the doubt, the vulnerability that exists in human life, and I have been impressed by how many thinkers in the literary, religious, and scientific stratospheres speak a similar language—Tolstoy, Thoreau, Tillich, Einstein, and others I cannot think of right now. As Einstein said, "He who can no longer wonder and stand rapt in awe, is as good as dead." Our real world often causes us to shun wonder and replace it with what is visible. When this happens, awe steps out of the picture.

Let me repeat those words: "He who can no longer wonder and stand rapt in awe, is as good as dead." Now, let us take a moment to examine this thing called *awe* a little more thoroughly. We talk of it a lot, but it is defined differently, I suspect, by each of us. Psychologist Dacher Keltner, director of the Berkeley Social Interaction Lab, defines awe as "the feeling of being in the presence of something vast or beyond human scale that transcends our current understanding of things."[5]

Dr. Keltner believes that the fact that we are wired to be able to experience awe makes us more cooperative because we realize we are all a small part of something much larger, which causes our thinking to shift from me to we. We are geared toward wanting to know what makes things tick; what is this thing beyond the thing we see? Being so wired, we search, hoping to glimpse something—even a vague idea of what is the impenetrable mystery. Perhaps part of this is motivated by the wish to act and believe as a part of *we* instead of *me.* We reach for that something that makes us feel a part of something much larger and more complete than ourselves.

Awe, or wonderment, is there when I experience those *ah-ha* moments: those times when a thought emerges from all thoughts and accosts me with what seem clarity and truth. We all have awesome moments, although we sometimes pass them off with a sigh or a shudder. I love to read something and think to myself, "What a great insight that is!" I read with a pen or pencil in hand to underline or make big Xs or stars by some concept that strikes me as profound. Or, have you ever taken a tape recorder while walking, hoping to grab any fleeting thought you might have?

I can speak only for myself, but if, like me, you regret not having the courage and insight in past years that you wish you might have had, give thanks that we have these latter days to add to our legacy, work toward a more peaceful world (if it may only be in our own senior home), look back on the experiences that may have given us a touch of wisdom, and ponder the great beyond. We do what we can.

Here is a good place for me to share another influence that has been important in my life. For many years I have had an e-mail relationship with a good friend who lives in Tehran. He has blessed my life with the rat-a-tat-tat of e-mails that have flown back and forth between us. Alirezza (Ali) teaches English and has visited the United States twice. He loves Americans and hates the divide that presently separates us. The stories he has shared with me from his Persian culture have broadened my thoughts. One story he recounted about his own convictions fits in quite well here.

Ali explains that there are two distinct interpretations of his faith. The first interpretation, under the influence of the Greek philosophers, relies mostly on the mind, reasoning, knowledge, and logic to find the way to God. The second considers inspiration and illumination of the heart from God as the best way to reach Him. grandfather was a dervish, a person who takes a vow of poverty and simplicity. Listen to this story he shared from Rumi's "Mathnavi":

> In a contest a king gave two opposite walls to two groups of people to paint to prove their mastery of painting and receive handsome rewards. They hung a curtain between the walls. As the first group of master painters was doing their best to bring their miraculous painting to completion on the first wall, the second group who did not even know how to paint started to clean and polish their wall. On the final day when the curtain was raised the king found the reflection of the painting on the clean and purified wall as beautiful as the original painting. This is the way of true dervishes. They are the ones who simplify their lives and purify their hearts to make a better "mirror" of themselves: one which reflects and not explains God's greatness and magnificence. Simple and pure. When I first heard Thoreau say, "Simplify, simplify," I cried.

Ali and I were brought together through the sharing of our love for Henry David Thoreau. My friend has translated Thoreau's *Walden* into Farsi in recent years, making it available for the first time to those who speak that language. He has always seen a connection between Thoreau and what I will call the poets of Persia: Rumi, Sufi, Hafiz, and others, and he sees similarities between what Thoreau taught and those things that were so important to his beloved dervish grandfather: love and simplicity. Does one find God through logic or love? Reason or inspiration? Science or mysticism? Do I need to explain what God is? Do I need to define Him? Do I need to make up doctrines about his wishes? No, says my friend. We simply try to mirror our inspiration as best we can—*just keep polishing ourselves.*

Ali's story left me realizing that until my last breath, what better life goal might I have than to strive to attempt to mirror what I see as God's wishes and goodness. I don't need to define God. I don't need to explain Him. I fear that my wall still has many blemishes, but perhaps I can use this ending time to try to become the person I would like to be, and do the things that I believe to be the will of God. I still need some polishing.

But let's go on. My friend, Emily Dickinson causes us to consider another avenue—faith:[6]

"Faith" is a fine invention
For Gentlemen who *see!*
But Microscopes are prudent
In an Emergency!

We can talk of awe, we can talk of creativity, and now, let's talk of faith. I have always wanted to mentally live in only one world and in that world, science and the spiritual must walk, if not hand-in-glove, then, at least, side by side. I'm not sure what Emily had in mind when she wrote this poem, but I like to assume that she would agree with me.

Our faith is "not a theoretical affirmation of something uncertain, it is the existential acceptance of something transcending ordinary experience"[7] wrote Paul Tillich. Tillich came into my life in a strange way: I discovered his tombstone on a visit to New Harmony, Indiana, a small town about twenty miles from where I was born in southern Indiana.

New Harmony is a most interesting place and well worth a visit because of its complex history and the philosophies that created it. It was built originally by the Rappites, or Harmonites, as a social attempt at religious communal living in the early 1800s, and then in the 1820s George Rapp, the founder, sold the property and the town to Robert Owen, a wealthy Scotsman. Owen led his group, known as the Boatload of Knowledge, down the Ohio River and then the Wabash River to this small town in an attempt to build a community based on universal education and philosophy, in which, as he saw it, the individual was submerged into the society. New Harmony is still there, the town and many of the early structures, but philosophically what remains today of these two attempts at the perfect society are the symbols of the beliefs of these two groups: I was intrigued by the Roofless Church, shaped like an upside-down rosebud, symbolizing that no roof, or barrier, should stand between religions; and I had to walk the labyrinth, built by the Rappites, symbolizing the many choices man must make in his life, and rewards for the proper selection; and finally, Paul Tillich Park, where Tillich's ashes were interred. Fascinated by what this small town symbolized, Tillich chose this spot for his personal memorial—a place that dreamed of bridging the thought process he endorsed between philosophy, theology, and technology.[8]

Yes, we all get our ideas and inspiration from this or that contact we may have had in life, and all I can tell you about my final look at life and death is dependent on what I have seen and heard in a long lifetime. It smacks of my experiences, experiences that may have meant little to me at the time I lived them, but gained importance when I rethought them later in my life.

We live with vulnerability and ambiguity throughout our life, as Brené Brown tells us, and as mentioned, particularly in our last years, we are tempted to push less hard against providence, letting someone else search, discover, and ponder, but after having taken care of all the practical aspects of living and not living, if we do not now look in the corners of our life and stand tall, when will we? Fright and caution and a limited perspective may cause us to let these years fly by with eyes shut and fearful of risk. If awe is replaced by fear, or shortsightedness, our vulnerability will stifle our courage. I had such a time in my own life.

When my mother died from Alzheimer's, instead of courage I felt anger. Instead of faith I felt alone. I turned away from any sense of awe or spiritual thought, feeling that there was no kindness in any God that would cause my dear mother such pain. It took me two years and the inner thought necessary to writing a book about Alzheimer's before I could once more stand rapt at the thought of that impenetrable something. Then one day it came, as many profound thoughts do, in the flash of a moment, and it came from a quote that suddenly made me take a deep breath and accept her death with a feeling of peace:

> What right have I to grieve who has not ceased to wonder. Only nature has a right to grieve perpetually, for she only is innocent. Soon the ice will melt, and the blackbirds sing along the river which he frequented, as pleasantly as ever. The same everlasting serenity will appear in this face of God, and we will not be sorrowful, if he is not.

This excerpt is from a letter dated March 2, 1842, written by Henry Thoreau to a Mrs. Lucy Brown. Thoreau's brother John had died in his arms of tetanus two months earlier.

I wonder if he could have ever realized what peace his words would leave in a heart like mine so many years later, causing me to suddenly find the humility to leave decisions of life and death to God—a God beyond the god of theism, a God who looks beyond life and death, a God beyond God that I newly discovered in this late moment of my life.

This was such an important moment in my life. I had found acceptance. I had found faith. I'm sure that others might have passed by Thoreau's words and found their own moment, but this was mine. I still remember taking a deep breath and feeling a heavy load lift from my heart. It's possible others might never feel the emotion that I did at that moment, at those words, but suddenly I became confident that I could trust such a God.

Somehow it felt right that I should hand over my grief to this higher power and finally have the *courage to be*—in spite of. In spite of not knowing, not understanding, not comprehending. At that moment I accepted the mystery. If God is not sorrowful at death, then He must not see the tragedy or even the finality in death that we do, and when I look at him in nature, the plan is there, the serenity is there, and I could accept what has been intended since the beginning of time. With that thought, and a lot of humility, I breathed a sigh of relief. I let God. No more need be said.

Social psychologist Paul Piff of the University of California, Irvine, says that "awe causes a kind of Be Here Now that seems to dissolve the self."[9]

It makes us act more generously, ethically, and fairly. And, in my case, it allowed me to hand my grief over to a higher power. All of this culminates for me in a single thought: If I can peacefully live my simple life, mirroring what appears to be the will of God, and creating what appears to be my designated work here on earth—my passions—I do believe I could say to myself, "You've done it, old girl. This is the *you* you can be proud to die with." Daring greatly and standing rapt with awe, facing ... who knows what, or whom?

I have to be careful, however. Living in this tentative world can make me impatient to find absolutes, and although I become very fond of my guesses, I have to remember: I am privy only to a mystery and to hints, viewpoints, and those special moments that each of us experiences. Realizing that my own tentative suppositions are only suggestions of ultimate truth, I can dare greatly and still be tolerant of another's conclusions, or should I say suppositions. Self-effacement encourages us to speak up, but at the same time listen with acceptance to ideas other than our own. A recognition of vulnerability and the uncertain nature of truth can make us more tolerant of others. In the roofless church of the world, all should be allowed to speak and search.

I am reminded of a definition of *truth* I read a few years ago in a book by Simon Blackburn called *Truth: A Guide* that helped me realize the unconfirmed nature of our individual opinions: If each of us were to shoot an arrow at a barn door, and then draw a circle around our personal arrow, saying with pride, "That's truth," in fact, which circle *is* absolute truth? We are privy to only hints, glimmers, and possibilities, so how can we say this or that is truth? One does not have to espouse relativism to look at things this way; in fact it is my way of celebrating inclusiveness.

In his book, Blackburn quotes Sir Francis Bacon:

> The human spirit (in its different dispositions in different men) is a variable thing, quite irregular, almost haphazard. Heraclitus well said that men seek knowledge in lesser, private worlds, not in the great or common world.[10]

What if we all shared our *what if* moments as part of a common world instead of getting hung up on our own individual truths? What if we all pooled our arrows and discovered that truth has many dimensions? What if all our thoughts and ideas are part of an Ultimate, and what if this Ultimate is far beyond our poor human knowledge? We may never find that our personal view is the right one or the only one, but let us have the courage to continue to search and examine the Being of Life. With courage we dare to search for truth, and we do it with a sense of wonderment and openness in our heart. These are the qualities I wish to treasure as I try to understand this bewildering universe I live in at this late stage of my life.

Today, I live with wonder at the eternal mystery of the universe. The question is, can I have the *courage to be,* to dare greatly, and to create and do, and find meaning in my present world in spite of that mystery? Here is where I need hope. With hope I am content to simply ponder, do my Being work by attempting to work toward peace, wisdom, and a positive legacy, as Dr. Thomas advised, and continue to look for the mystery that is.

In so doing we have to work with the me that so long ago came from the everywhere into the here. Remember the song "Trouble" from a few years back? The lyrics are easy to remember, something like "trouble, trouble, trouble ... worry, worry, worry."[11] I tend to fret and worry, hence I sit and write to help me gain control over these emotions that make life difficult. Yes, life is precarious and precious, but seldom does worry change the outcome. And if God does not worry, why should I? Somewhere out there is "the plan," and as the saying goes, "it is well beyond my pay grade."

I wish I could introduce you to all the older persons I have met who deal with age and productivity well, but let me introduce you, in this final chapter, to my friend A. I have a friend here at Planet X who in his pre-stroke life was a recognized artist in the East. My friend may worry, as I do, but he deals with hope with a very wry sense of humor. He has told me of his youthful summers working and traveling with a carnival, and with a sense of humor unparalleled he describes his first love—in kindergarten.

Yesterday I interrupted his TV ball game and we talked. I told him how I admire his ability to deal with his very serious stroke and still go out with his caregiver and sit in the car and continue to paint. (He signs his later work with his name and PS—Post Stroke—which shows both his humor and his acceptance of what has happened to him.) In our conversation I mentioned how I love the way he has used his humor to help him accept his present condition, and with a graceful fling of his hands he smiled, got a twinkle in his eye, and said, "Humor in tragedy," as though he were naming a painting. PS: His humor and his indomitable spirit have helped A. continue to hope, to do, and to accept what is.

Looking at hope as a quest beacon to guide this part of my life as fully as I am able, I have to ask: what am I pursuing? I have really enjoyed my old age, and yet, looking ahead to the end of life does not send me into raptures. As far as I know, few come back to tell us what to expect. I have talked to a few friends here at Planet X who are ready to die. I don't know if I will come to this resigned state anytime soon, but right now I am enjoying my life, and as Robert Frost said, I feel I have "miles to go before I sleep."[12] I'm already thinking about possible books four and five, and yet I have accepted the idea that I am not in charge of when I am to leave this present world. My research tells me there are many things I can do that may extend my time here, and we do what we can. But ultimately my life rests in hands other than mine.

One way I see to thwart death is to go leaving nothing behind that I wish to do. In the past, the way I considered death, and really, how most people consider death, was to not consider it. "This isn't going to happen to me, at least not for a very, very, very long time." Well, now I'm eighty-five. Yes, ladies and gentlemen, this *is* going to happen. And then I remember a quote from Viktor Frankl, wherein he quotes the philosopher Friedrich Nietzsche: "Those who have a 'why' to live, can bear with almost any 'how.'"[13]

I am sure that one important thing I need to do is to reflect on what I've done in my life. This last act of reflection demands that I be open and honest with myself. Perhaps I will even have time to undo some mistakes. What motivates us in this stage of our lives? What is it that sets this time apart from the difficult times that have come before? It is that this is our final time, and we know it, and what we do is final.

Yes, yes, I can accept the reflection in the mirror and the many signs of aging that accompany it. But can I also move on and continue to create, to smile, to learn, and to teach? What do I need to keep me strong and supplied with the *courage to be* that Tillich talks about?

Shortly after we moved to Planet X, a dove or pigeon (we never decided which) also decided to move here. She set up housekeeping on the ledge outside the window we all passed on the way to and from meals. She was white with a cocoa brown touch to her wings, and from the first she would show up at dusk and spend the night cuddled by our window. She would watch as we waved at her, and we named her Hope.

We all looked for Hope, and she never failed us. She would come at about seven each evening, rain, hail, or snow, and seemed to say hello to us through the window as we trailed back from dinner. I even imagined that she liked being close to other beings and pitied her when the weather was cold—she who must remain on her small shelf, while I was snug and warm within.

Hope left us one day and never returned. She had been there for at least a year's full of nights, and then we had to live our nights without her. Was Hope gone? Did we no longer have Hope? Our physical world, as in so many instances, had teased us and given us a pleasant metaphor, but never showed us the real meaning of this four-letter word. Still, a year later, as I pass that window, I still hope—hope that she might return. Hope is a feeling of trust that if Hope is gone, there is still hope. It is having trust, in spite of everything. For me, it is part of the *courage to be.*

Ironically, this is true so many times in this human life: now that Hope is gone, all we have is hope. Perhaps Hope was trying to give us something: hope that lonely little bird might have been a messenger of life itself. And with this hope there is awe in the unknown. We are here and then we are gone. We know not what or where, but we hope. We don't know if we will be able to leave a legacy, but we hope.

And then it comes. Death. As I look back on my father's final illness when he was seventy-nine, I realize I learned something about hope from him. He had developed pain in his left cheek that refused to go away, and a trip to a specialist and a biopsy revealed a squamous cell cancer in his sinus and cheek. Part of the bone had already been consumed, and there was no way to remove the evil thing.

"Doc, I'm not afraid to live and I'm not afraid to die, but what about the pain?" my father asked.

The doctor quietly explained the situation and offered radiation and chemotherapy as stopgap measures, telling my father that such treatments might make his death less painful. The doctor said he could expect about twenty-four months and that during the last months hospice would provide palliative care for any pain he might have.

My father followed the doctor's advice and had a few weeks of radiation treatments and chemo trips to the hospital, and then he became ever weaker and quieter. He could do little, and he had some pain, but to this day I can see him sitting on the back porch weaving baskets; it was something he could still enjoy doing, now that standing at his beloved workbench was too tiring for him. My heart broke every time I saw him sitting there, and yet, he lived and he worked and he never complained. I learned that in death we have choices, too. He chose to be courageous.

Soon the doctor said he had done all he could and suggested we call hospice. The hospice nurse came and gave Mother all the reading material that explained that hospice provided palliative care only and was a service for those who had a short time to live. Mother rebelled.

"We'll keep fighting. We'll find another doctor," she demanded. "I don't like to give up like this." This said with all the tears in the world.

"No." My father interrupted. "There is a time to live and a time to die. This is that time."

We don't choose when to die, or what will take us, but we can choose to accept the inevitable with hope and peace. It's our job—it is part of the *courage to be.*

I thought my heart would burst with grief. Deep down, I didn't want to accept that it was my father's time, but I shed tears of pride as I thought of his response. The death time will come to all of us, and I only hope I can approach it with the courage and acceptance of my father.

I held Dad's arm as he was dying and felt his pulse, and I stayed in that spot until I felt it no more. At one point my father looked at me, and his eyes grew wide and then wider, as he partially lifted himself off the bed. I have always wondered what he was trying to say and what he was seeing. And then, with one last pulse beat, he was gone. I could no longer ask him for advice, or feel his love as he would walk by and pull my ear. My father was no longer reachable. This body, this object that remained, was only a shell. My father was no longer there. I finally realized that we only borrow this body, and we aren't in charge of when or where it will no longer be needed. The real us is more than our body, but what it is, is still an unknown. As I look back I must concede: if God is at peace, why should I not be as well? My father no longer inhabited this frame. Where had my father's spirit, his energy gone? Energy doesn't die, science has told us. I wondered. I hoped.

Some of us deal with death more efficiently and calmly than others. Some of us have profound belief systems with which to deal with the inevitable, while others wonder and wander. I remember my grandmother's words when my great-grandmother died: "I wonder how those who don't believe that they'll see their loved ones again ever deal with death?" With faith or without it, wondering and hoping, death must be dealt with.

My friend K. told us she saw her deceased husband quite often. She heard him playing the piano and felt him touch her in the night, and she was comforted. He had been gone for some time, but he continued to call her to him. "I'm ready to go to F.," she told me calmly. "He wants me to be with him."

A few weeks ago, K. went home to her beloved husband. Now both are at peace. I wonder if he asked her, "What took you so long?" This faith in a life after death with those we love can be tied to a belief system, or it can be sensed with the soul. One of my friends saw the afterlife in this way: "If there is no life after death, there is no justice." I've often thought this. Justice is a concept in this life, but is it eternal? I don't know. No one does.

I remember so vividly what I witnessed at my father's death, being so close to the body as it rid itself of human life. My father's individuality, his energy, and his love were no longer in the body. They had fled, and what was left was not my father.

Daring and courage become harder to bring forth the weaker we become. High-minded thoughts are fine, but bravery in the face of finality is difficult. We can be brash and terribly confident if we are healthy. It is easy to be enthusiastic, wise, and active, even in old age, if health is on our side. But to become ill and spend time in the hospital, or in an assisted living or a nursing home, and have the life gradually seep from us can lead to depression, anger, or even a desire to quit and be done with it all. Add to this the effect this has on others. Here at Planet X we have had several stroke and heart attack victims this winter. Two were my very good friends, and their deaths were extremely hard on their families and friends.

In a way, my mother's Alzheimer's protected her from thinking about death. I believe for her that was a blessing, for she had feared death dreadfully. Perhaps God in His mercy took away her fears in this way. She entered a comatose state for about a week before she died, and then passed as we all would like to, in her sleep. Death had become very real to me at my father's passing, and then even more real when Mother died. Suddenly there was no generation between me and the grave. Now it was my time to think beyond.

We have talked about how aging is not a disease. Nevertheless, the human body does become less muscular and loses nutrients and antioxidants as it grows old. Our cells do not reproduce as before. Yes, we can hopefully keep ourselves active by watching our habits. But then, death comes. The body we have borrowed, regardless of our patient care, at last gives in. And then what? It bothers me to think that I won't be a part of what will happen next in this life. I guess I'm just terribly meddlesome. I don't like to think I can't have a cup of coffee, read the newspaper, listen to TV, and ask my kids how they're doing. And what if I can never go to Walmart again? What a tragedy.

Although I don't know what happens next, I do know that my parents are still with me in some ways. I remember so many things they taught me. So many shared experiences. So much love. Good memories are a wonderful legacy, but they are often guaranteed to bring forth tears. I only hope that I have left my own children with memories that will feed their hearts and souls. I know I envision both of my parents as links in my personal chain of love and wisdom.

How lucky I am to have had my life, and to have such good memories—such moorings. I only hope I can leave as rich a legacy. I know that if I can approach my aging with thought, with awe, and with courage, I will be more likely to leave a legacy I can be proud of. Don't be afraid of aging. Dare greatly, and then fall to your knees.

So, what about the rest of our life? Dr. George Vaillant of Harvard Medical School says that the Harvard Study of Adult Behavior revealed two pillars of happiness in life: "One is love, the other is finding a way of coping with life that does not push love away."[14] And then we have the words of Viktor Frankl: "Love is the ultimate bestower of meaning."[15] We may ask ourselves, where did this gift of love come from?

> The snow falls on no two trees alike, but the forms it assumes are as various as those of the twigs and leaves which receive it. They are, as it were, pre-determined by the genius of the tree. So one divine spirit descends alike on all, but bears a peculiar fruit in each.... I look under the lids of Time.
> —Henry David Thoreau, Journal, January 30, 1841

And so, finally, just like Mary Lee Bendolph, the quilter from Gee's Bend, we come to the place where we all eventually arrive: the spirit, the mystery, and the God beyond God. Again I turn to the poetic, and my favorite poet, Mary Oliver, in "Mysteries, Yes":

> Let me keep company always with those who say
> "Look!" and laugh in astonishment,
> and bow their heads.

Last night I went to sleep with all these thoughts whirling in my brain, and I awoke this morning with the unsettled feeling that I had to finish a crossword puzzle I had been working on in my dream. I had one word left, but as I looked about in my dream for the list of clues, I discovered it was missing. I searched and searched, but there were no clues anywhere I looked. There sat the incomplete puzzle, waiting for me to find the last answer, and I had no clue! I believe my dream was showing me, in a way I could understand, that I was too human, too unknowing to have the secret of that final word—that I could only awaken from my dream and stand in awe.

> Time is but the stream I go a-fishing in. I drink at it; but while I drink I see the sandy bottom and detect how shallow it is. Its thin current slides away, but eternity remains. I would drink deeper; fish in the sky, whose bottom is pebbly with stars.
>
> —Henry David Thoreau, *Walden*

I would fish in the stars. But wait! Today's a new day! And the best thing I can be doing, as I complete this life, is to look my age, myself, and my life squarely in the eye: Here you are, you silly old fool. You're still above ground, aren't you? Well, then, act like it! Do something! Take your courage in hand and live and love! Life is good. Can death not be as well? Let the mystery remain the mystery.

> Life should not be a journey to the grave with the intention of arriving safely in a pretty and well preserved body, but rather to skid in broadside in a cloud of smoke, thoroughly used up, totally worn out, and loudly proclaiming "Wow! What a Ride!"
>
> —Hunter S. Thompson, *The Proud Highway*

Full stop.

Notes

PREFACE

1. Robert N. Butler, *Why Survive? Being Old in America* (Baltimore: Johns Hopkins University Press, 1975).

ONE

1. Natalie O'Donnell Wood. "Colorado's Budget Faces Immediate Pressure from Changing Demographics," December 16, 2016, accessed July 13, 2017, http:// www.bellpolicy.org/research/colorados-budget-faces-immediate-pressure-chang ing-demographics.
2. US Government Accountability Office, "Retirement Security: Most Households Approaching Retirement Have Low Savings" (GAO-15-419), May 12, 2015, https://www.gao.gov/products/GAO-15-419.
3. Ruth Bennett and Judith Eckman, "Attitudes toward Aging: A Critical Examination of Recent Literature and Implications for Future Research," in *The Psychology of Adult Development and Aging,* ed. Carol Eisendorfer and Lawton M. Powell (Washington, DC: American Psychological Association, 1973), 575–97. An abstract for this chapter is available at https://doi.org/10.1037/10044-018.
4. Ibid.
5. American Psychological Association, *Aging and Depression,* accessed July 13, 2017, http://www.apa.org/helpcenter/aging-depression.aspx.
6. Carmen DeNavas and Bernadette D. Proctor, *Income and Poverty in the United States: 2014* (Washington, DC: US Census Bureau, 2015), https://www.census .gov/content/dam/Census/library/publications/2015/demo/p60-252.pdf.
7. Encarnacion Pyle, "Ohio's Elderly Forced to Choose between Food or Medicine," *Columbus Dispatch,* May 3, 2015, http://www.dispatch.com/article/20150503/NE WS/305039917.

TWO

1. Jill McCorkle, *Life after Life* (Chapel Hill, NC: Algonquin Books, 2013).
2. Gay Hanna and Susan Perlstein, *Creativity Matters: Arts and Aging in America,*

Americans for the Arts Monograph Series (Washington, DC: Americans for the Arts, 2008), https://www.giarts.org/sites/default/files/Monograph_Creativity-Matters-Arts-and-Aging-in-America.pdf.

THREE

1. Karl Vick, "The Home of the Future," *Time,* March 23, 2017, http://time.com/4710619/the-home-of-the-future/

FOUR

1. Among others, the Harvard Study of Adult Development (http://www.adultdevelopmentstudy.org/), which we will talk about in chapter 6, heavily supports this.

FIVE

1. Joan Chittister, *The Gift of Years* (New York: Blue Bridge Publishing, 2008).
2. Chapter 6 is where we really talk about research. Two good articles are "The Secrets of Aging Well" from *WebMD* and Liz Mineo's "Good Genes are Nice, But Joy Is Better," both listed in the bibliography.

SIX

1. Carolyn Gregoire, "This Man Faced Unimaginable Suffering," *Huffington Post,* April 2, 2014, http://www.huffingtonpost.com/2014/02/04/this-book-youve-probably-_n_4705123.html.
2. Syphilis was very common in the powdered wig era and the wigs were often used to cover the loss of hair that victims suffered. For a history of American attitudes toward againg, see David H. Fischer, *Growing Old in America* (New York: Oxford University Press, 1977).
3. Eric Lindland, Marissa Fond, Abigail Haydon, and Nathaniel Kendall-Taylor, *Gauging Aging: Mapping the Gaps between Expert and Public Understandings of Aging in America* (Washington, DC: Frameworks Institute, 2015). https://frameworksinstitute.org/assets/files/aging_mtg.pdf.
4. American Federation for Aging Research (AFAR), *Gauging Aging: Report on Public Perception of Aging,* accessed July 13, 2017, https://www.afar.org/gauging-aging-report-on-public-perception-of-aging/.
5. Ibid.
6. This ninth stage is experienced in the eighties and nineties and is accompanied by a loss of physical health, friends, family members, and independence, in addition to

isolation from society. Often during this time, individuals are put into retirement communities and assisted living facilities, which Joan viewed as isolating them from society and from youth. Of course, she was writing at a time when such residences were considered "holding pens."

Joan Erikson's quote is from *Wikipedia,* s.v. "Joan Erikson," last modified February 17, 2017, https://en.wikipedia.org/wiki/Joan_Erikson. The original source is identified as Daniel Benveniste, "The Importance of Play in Adulthood: A Dialogue with Joan Erikson," *The Psychoanalytic Study of the Child* 53.

7. Daniel Goleman, "Erikson, in His Own Old Age, Expands His View of Life," *New York Times,* June 14, 1988, http://www.nytimes.com/books/99/08/22/specials/erikson-old.html.

8. A great resource for guided autobiography is http://guidedautobiography.com. From the website ("About Us," http://guidedautobiography.com/guided-autobiography/):

"Guided Autobiography (GAB) has been researched and developed by Dr. James Birren over the past 40 years as a method for helping people document their life stories.... Writing and sharing life stories with others is an ideal way to find new meaning in life and to put life events into perspective. While connecting with one another on their journeys of self-discovery, participants feel enlivened by the group experience and gain a greater appreciation of their own lives and of the lives of others. GAB can be a powerful catalyst for improved self-esteem, self-confidence and communication within communities and within families.

"Some of the benefits of GAB include:
- Increased self-acceptance
- Decreased anxiety and tension
- Increased energy and vigor
- Increased positive view of others
- A feeling of connectedness and friendship"

9. David Halberstam, "A Modest Generation," *Harvard Magazine,* May/June 2005, http://harvardmagazine.com/2005/05/a-modest-generation.html.

10. George Packer, *David Halberstam Obituary,* Postscript, *New Yorker,* May 7, 2007, http://www.newyorker.com/magazine/2007/05/07/david-halberstam.

11. Sherwin B. Nuland, *The Art of Aging: A Doctor's Prescription for Well-Being* (New York: Random House, 2008).

12. Kennedy's records have since been closed until the year 2040.

13. "The Secrets of Aging Well: Live Long and Prosper," *WebMD,* 2002, accessed July 13, 2017, http://www.webmd.com/healthy-aging/features/secrets-of-aging-well#1.

14. Scott Stossel, "What Makes Us Happy, Revisited," *Atlantic,* May 2013, https://www .theatlantic.com/magazine/archive/2013/05/thanks-mom/309287/. *(Emphasis mine.)*

15. Liz Mineo, "Good Genes Are Nice, But Joy Is Better," *Harvard Gazette,* April, 11, 2017, http://news.harvard.edu/gazette/story/2017/04/over-nearly-80-years-harvard-study-has-been-showing-how-to-live-a-healthy-and-happy-life/. *(Emphasis mine.)*

16. Robert Waldinger, "What Makes a Good Life? Lessons from the Longest Study on Happiness," TED video, accessed July 13, 2017, https://www.ted.com/talks /robert_waldinger_what_makes_a_good_life_lessons_from_the_longest_study _on_happiness/transcript?language=en.

17. "The Secrets of Aging Well: Live Long and Prosper." *(Emphasis mine.)*

18. Ibid.

19. http://www.edenalt.org/. The philosophy originally began in nursing homes and now has three versions, from nursing home care to care in the home.

20. *Eden Alternative: It Can Be Different!,* accessed July 13, 2017, http://www.edenalt .org/wordpress/wp-content/uploads/2014/02/Eden_Overview_092613LR.pdf.

21. A good place to start is the "About" page: http://www.edenalt.org/about-the-eden -alternative/.

22. William H. Thomas, *What Are Old People For? (Emphasis mine.)*

23. Ibid.

24. Paula Span, "Living on Purpose," The New Old Age Blog, *New York Times,* June 3, 2014, https://newoldage.blogs.nytimes.com/2014/6/03/living-on-purpose/.

25. Ibid. *(Emphasis mine.)*

26. Ibid.

27. "Sense of Purpose in Life Linked to Lower Mortality and Cardiovascular Risk," *ScienceDaily,* December 3, 2015, accessed June 1, 2017, www.sciencedaily.com/re leases/2015/12/151203112844.htm.

28. Amy Dickinson, Dear Amy, *Chicago Tribune,* November 4, 2014, http://www.chica gotribune.com/lifestyles/askamy/ct-daughter-has-bisexual-boyfriend-20141102 -column.html. It's the lovely letter from *Grateful for More Chances.*

29. Melinda Beck, "Starting to Feel Older? New Studies Show Attitude Can Be Critical," Heath Matters, *Wall Street Journal,* updated October 17, 2009. https://www .wsj.com/articles/SB10001424052748704471504574445263666118226.

30. Ibid.

31. Camille Peri, "What I Wish I'd Known About 'Elderspeak': Psychologist Becca Levy; What a Yale Professor Learned about the Way We Think about and Talk to the Elderly," accessed July 13, 2017, https://www.caring.com/reflections/becca -levy-reflection.

32. John Leland, "In 'Sweetie' and 'Dear,' a Hurt for the Elderly," *New York Times,* October 6, 2008, http://www.nytimes.com/2008/10/07/us/07aging.html. *(Emphasis mine.)*

33. Lea Winerman, "A Healthy Mind, a Longer Life," *Monitor* 37, no. 10 (2006): 42, http://www.apa.org/monitor/nov06/healthy.aspx. *(Emphasis mine.)*

34. Becca R. Levy, "Mind Matters: Cognitive and Physical Effects of Aging Self-Stereotypes," *Journal of Gerontology: Psychological Sciences* 58, no. 4 (2003): P20–P211, https://doi.org/10.1093/geronb/58.4.P203.

35. Lea Winerman, "A Healthy Mind, a Longer Life."

36. Anna Azvolinsky, "Protein Protects Aging Brain," Daily News, *The Scientist,* March 19, 2014. http://www.the-scientist.com/?articles.view/articleNo/39492/title/Protein-Protects-Aging-Brain/.

37. Sherwin B. Nuland, *The Art of Aging.*

38. Anna Azvolinsky, "Protein Protects Aging Brain."

39. Dan Buettner, *The Blue Zones: Lessons for Living Longer from the People Who've Lived the Longest* (Washington, DC: National Geographic Society, 2010).

40. Sherwin B. Nuland, *The Art of Aging.*

41. Carolyn Gregoire, "This Man Faced Unimaginable Suffering."

SEVEN

1. Paulo Coelho, *The Alchemist,* trans. Alan R. Clarke (New York: Harper One, 1993).

2. *Peepmobile* is a name I use for the motorized scooters and wheelchairs that some residents are forced to use. I really would love to ride in one of those three-wheeled scooters. The only problem is that they can go pretty fast and I would probably smack into a wall somewhere!

3. Laura L. Carstensen et al., "Emotional Experience Improves with Age: Evidence Based on Over 10 Years of Experience Sampling," *Psychology and Aging* 26, no. 1 (2011): 21–33, http://dx.doi.org/10.1037/a0021285. This article is freely available at https://www.ncbi.nlm.nih.gov/pmc/articles/PMC3332527/.

4. Ibid.

EIGHT

1. Jonathan Safron Foer, *Here I Am* (New York: Farrar, Straus and Giroux, 2016).

2. William Powers, *Hamlet's BlackBerry* (New York: HarperCollins, 2010).

3. Gay Hanna and Susan Perlstein, *Creativity Matters: Arts and Aging in America,* Americans for the Arts Monograph Series (Washington, DC: Americans for the Arts, 2008), https://www.giarts.org/sites/default/files/Monograph_Creativity-Matters-Arts-and-Aging-in-America.pdf.

4. Nohl Martin Fouroohi and Ellen Liu Kellor, "Creativity, Activity, and Longevity," *New LifeStyles Senior Industry Blog,* April 2, 2006, accessed July 13, 2017, https://www.newlifestyles.com/blog/posts/2006/04/Creativity-Activity-and-Longevity.

5. Gay Hanna and Susan Perlstein, *Creativity Matters.*

6. Robert N. Butler, *Why Survive? Being Old in America* (Baltimore: Johns Hopkins University Press, 1975).

7. "MIM Art Program," accessed July 14, 2017, http://www.alz.org/co/in_my_community_art_program.asp.

8. René Laforestrie, *L'âge de Créer* (London: Centurion Press, 1991).

9. Ibid.

10. Douglas Hofstadter, *Gödel, Escher, Bach* (New York: Basic Books, 1999).

    Here, Dr. Hofstadter says it in a different way: "I guess I'm the type for whom analogy is the driving force behind the way I think. And I've managed to convince myself that analogy is really at the core of thinking—not just for myself, but for other people, too. I'm trying to put forth a vision of thought that involves—if you don't want to say 'analogy-making' you can say 'stripping away irrelevancies to get at the gist of things.' I feel I've discovered something essential about what thinking is, and I'm on a crusade to make it clear to everybody." This is from a 1995 interview of Dr. Hofstadter: "By Analogy: A Talk with the Most Remarkable Researcher in Artificial Intelligence Today, Douglas Hofstadter, the Author of Gödel, Escher, Bach," *Wired,* November 1, 1995, https://www.wired.com/1995/11/kelly/.

11. Claire Martin, "Aging Well Begins with Being Active, Social and Consciously Contributing to Your Community," *Denver Post,* March 21, 2014, updated April 27, 2016, http://www.denverpost.com/2014/03/21/aging-well-begins-with-being-active-social-and-consciously-contributing-to-your-community/.

12. Allen Weiss, "Mindfulness: Paying Attention to What's Really Important," accessed July 5, 2017, https://www.agingcare.com/articles/mindfulness-paying-attention-to-whats-important-175242.htm.

13. William H. Thomas, *What Are Old People For? How Elders Will Save the World,* (St. Louis: VanderWyk & Burnham, 2007).

14. Ibid.

15. Ibid.

16. Ibid.

17. Michael Ramscar et al., "The Myth of Cognitive Decline: Non-Linear Dynamics of Lifelong Learning," *Topics in Cognitive Science,* January 13, 2014, https://doi.org/10.1111/tops.12078.

18. Zalman Schachter-Shalomi and Ronald S. Miller, *From Age-ing to Sage-ing: A Revolutionary Approach to Growing Older* (New York: Time Warner Books, 1997).

NINE

1. Brené Brown, *Daring Greatly: How the Courage to Be Vulnerable Transforms the Way We Live, Love, Parent, and Lead* (New York: Avery, 2012).
2. "The World As I See It: An Essay by Einstein," accessed July 18, 2017, http://histo ry.aip.org/history/exhibits/einstein/essay.htm.
3. Scholars differ greatly in their view of Einstein's religion. Some see him as a pantheist and some believe that he did not believe in God. Obviously his view of any God or First Cause was beyond the theological viewpoint.
4. Paul Tillich, *The Courage to Be* (New Haven: Yale University Press, 1952).
5. Paula Spencer Scott, "Feeling Awe May Be the Secret to Health and Happiness," *Parade,* October, 9, 2016, https://parade.com/513786/paulaspencer/feeling-awe -may-be-the-secret-to-health-and-happiness/.
6. Source: *The Poems of Emily Dickinson: Reading Edition,* edited by Ralph W. Franklin, Cambridge, Mass.: The Belknap Press of Harvard University Press, Copyright © 1998, 1999 by the President and Fellows of Harvard College. Copyright © 1951, 1955, 1979, 1983 by the President and Fellows of Harvard College.
7. Paul Tillich, *The Courage to Be.*
8. Don Blair, *The New Harmony Story* (New Harmony, IN: New Harmony Publications Committee, n.d.).
9. Paula Spencer Scott, "Feeling Awe May Be the Secret to Health and Happiness."
10. Simon Blackburn, *Truth: A Guide* (London: Oxford University Press, 2005).
11. I'm recalling it from the Travelers Insurance commercial of a few years ago with the cute dog. The song was written and performed by Ray LaMontagne.
12. From the poem "Stopping by Woods on a Snowy Evening."
13. Paula Spencer Scott, "Feeling Awe May Be the Secret to Health and Happiness."
14. Carolyn Gregoire, "This Man Faced Unimaginable Suffering," *Huffington Post,* April 2, 2014, http://www.huffingtonpost.com/2014/02/04/this-book-youve-prob ably-_n_4705123.html.
15. From his book *Man's Search for Meaning.*

Bibliography

Alzheimer's Association. "MIM Art Program." http://www.alz.org/co/in_my_commu nity_art_program.asp.

American Federation for Aging Research (AFAR). "Gauging Aging: Report on Public Perception of Aging." Accessed July 13, 2017. https://www.afar.org/gaug ing-aging-report-on-public-perception-of-aging.

American Psychological Association. "Aging and Depression." Accessed July 13, 2017. http://www.apa.org/helpcenter/aging-depression.aspx.

Azvolinsky, Anna. "Protein Protects Aging Brain." Daily News, *The Scientist,* March 19, 2014. http://www.the-scientist.com/?articles.view/articleNo/39492 /title/Protein-Protects-Aging-Brain/.

Beck, Melinda. "Starting to Feel Older? New Studies Show Attitude Can Be Critical." Heath Matters, *Wall Street Journal.* Updated October 17, 2009. https://www.wsj.com /articles/SB10001424052748704471504574445263666118226.

Bennett, Ruth, and Judith Eckman. "Attitudes toward Aging: A Critical Examination of Recent Literature and Implications for Future Research." In *The Psychology of Adult Development and Aging,* edited by Carol Eisendorfer and Lawton M. Powell, 575–97. Washington, DC: American Psychological Association, 1973.

Blackburn, Simon. *Truth: A Guide.* London: Oxford University Press, 2005.

Blair, Don. *The New Harmony Story.* New Harmony, IN: New Harmony Publications Committee, n.d.

Brown, Brené. *Daring Greatly: How the Courage to Be Vulnerable Transforms the Way We Live, Love, Parent, and Lead.* New York: Avery, 2012.

Buettner, Dan. *The Blue Zones: Lessons for Living Longer from the People Who've Lived the Longest.* Washington, DC: National Geographic Society, 2010.

Butler, Robert N. *Why Survive? Being Old in America.* Baltimore: Johns Hopkins University Press, 1975.

"By Analogy: A Talk with the Most Remarkable Researcher in Artificial Intelligence Today, Douglas Hofstadter, the Author of Gödel, Escher, Bach." *Wired,* November 1, 1995. https://www.wired.com/1995/11/kelly/.

Carstensen, Laura L., Bulent Turan, Susanne Scheibe, Nilam Ram, Hal Ersner-Hershfield, Gregory R. Samanez-Larkin, Kathryn P. Brooks, and John R. Nesselroade. "Emotional Experience Improves with Age: Evidence Based on Over 10 Years of Experience Sampling." *Psychology and Aging* 26, no. 1 (2011): 21–33, https://doi.org/10.1037/a0021285.

Chittister, Joan. *The Gift of Years.* New York: Blue Bridge Publishing, 2008.

Coelho, Paulo. *The Alchemist.* Translated by Alan R. Clarke. New York: Harper One, 1993.

DeNavas-Walt, Carmen, and Bernadette D. Proctor. *Income and Poverty in the United States: 2014.* Washington, DC: US Census Bureau, 2015. https://www.census.gov/content/dam/Census/library/publications/2015/demo/p60-252.pdf.

Eden Alternative: It Can Be Different! Accessed July 13, 2017. http://www.edenalt.org/wordpress/wp-content/uploads/2014/02/Eden_Over view_092613LR.pdf.

Fischer, David H. *Growing Old in America.* New York: Oxford University Press, 1977.

Foer, Jonathan Safron. *Here I Am.* New York: Farrar, Straus and Giroux, 2016.

Fouroohi, Nohl Martin, and Ellen Liu Kellor. "Creativity, Activity, and Longevity." *New LifeStyles Senior Industry Blog,* April 2, 2006. Accessed July 13, 2017. https://www.newlifestyles.com/blog/posts/2006/04/Creativity-Activity-and-Longevity.

Goleman, Daniel. "Erikson, in His Own Old Age, Expands His View of Life." *New York Times,* June 14, 1988. http://www.nytimes.com/books/99/08/22/specials/erikson-old.html

Gregoire, Carolyn. "This Man Faced Unimaginable Suffering." *The Huffington Post,* April 2, 2014. http://www.huffingtonpost.com/2014/02/04/this-book-youve-probably-_n_4705123.html.

Halberstam, David. "A Modest Generation." *Harvard Magazine,* May/June 2005. http://harvardmagazine.com/2005/05/a-modest-generation.html.

Hanna, Gay, and Susan Perlstein. *Creativity Matters: Arts and Aging in America.* Americans for the Arts Monograph Series. Washington, DC: Americans for the Arts, 2008. https://www.giarts.org/sites/default/files/Monograph_Creativity-Matters-Arts-and-Aging-in-America.pdf.

Hofstadter, Douglas. *Gödel, Escher, Bach.* New York: Basic Books, 1999.

Kim, Sin-Hyang, and Sihyun Park, "A Meta-Analysis of the Correlates of Successful Aging in Older Adults, *Research on Aging* 39, no. 5 (2017). https://doi.org/10.1177/0164027516656040

Laforestrie, René. *L'âge de Créer.* London: Centurion Press, 1991.

Leland, John. "In 'Sweetie' and 'Dear,' a Hurt for the Elderly. *New York Times,* October 6, 2008. http://www.nytimes.com/2008/10/07/us/07aging.html.